Dr. Michael Berglund takes a holistic, nutritionally, ...ed approach to hormone imbalances and fatigue-related issues, including thyroid and adrenal dysfunctions. His well-written book provides a comprehensive holistic approach to the hormone imbalances that cause fatigue, and it encourages us to address and resolve the underlying causes rather than mask symptoms. In a clear, compassionate tone, Dr. Berglund explains why and how safer, natural treatments with the fewest side effects are usually preferable to more aggressive treatments typically offered by conventional medicine. Dr. Berglund's book makes a valuable contribution to our ongoing and expanding discussion of the diagnosis and treatment of thyroid, adrenal, and other hormonal imbalances.

—MARY SHOMON
THYROID PATIENT ADVOCATE AND *NEW YORK TIMES*
BEST-SELLING AUTHOR OF *THE THYROID DIET*

I know many Christians who live with chronic pain, immune disorders, and other health problems, and they rarely feel that a medical professional understands their issues. In fact, some doctors seem out of touch with how God designed the body to function, so they only prescribe medications rather than dealing with root causes of illness. I am so thankful for a man like Michael Berglund, who has integrated his Christian faith into his career as a health professional. Michael combines his medical training with plenty of practical advice as well as solid spiritual counsel. You will be refreshed while reading this book—and if you follow the author's advice, I also believe you will feel better!

—J. LEE GRADY
AUTHOR, MINISTER, AND FORMER EDITOR
OF *CHARISMA* MAGAZINE

TIRED OF BEING
SICK
AND
TIRED

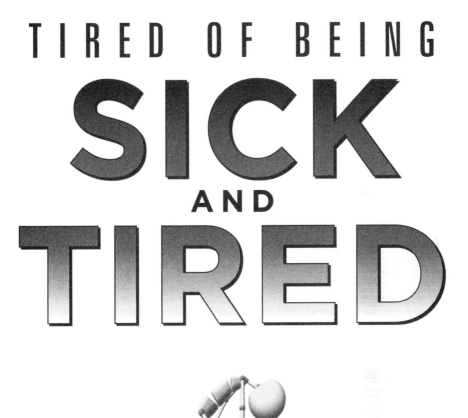

MICHAEL BERGLUND, DC

CHARISMA
HOUSE

Most CHARISMA HOUSE BOOK GROUP products are available at special quantity discounts for bulk purchase for sales promotions, premiums, fund-raising, and educational needs. For details, write Charisma House Book Group, 600 Rinehart Road, Lake Mary, Florida 32746, or telephone (407) 333-0600.

TIRED OF BEING SICK AND TIRED by Michael Berglund
Published by Siloam
Charisma Media/Charisma House Book Group
600 Rinehart Road
Lake Mary, Florida 32746
www.charismahouse.com

Unless otherwise noted, all Scripture quotations are from the New American Standard Bible, Copyright © 1960, 1962, 1963, 1968, 1971, 1972, 1973, 1975, 1977, 1995 by The Lockman Foundation. Used by permission. (www.Lockman.org)

Scripture quotations marked ESV are from the Holy Bible, English Standard Version. Copyright © 2001 by Crossway Bibles, a division of Good News Publishers. Used by permission.

Scripture quotations marked KJV are from the King James Version of the Bible.

Scripture quotations marked NIV are from the Holy Bible, New International Version. Copyright © 1973, 1978, 1984, International Bible Society. Used by permission.

Cover design by Justin Evans
Design Director: Bill Johnson

Visit the author's website at www.berglundcenter.com.

Library of Congress Cataloging-in-Publication Data
Berglund, Michael.
  Tired of being sick and tired / Michael Berglund.
    p. cm.
  Includes bibliographical references (p.   ) and index.
  ISBN 978-1-61638-467-8 (trade paper) -- ISBN 978-1-61638-577-4
  (e-book) 1. Thyroid gland--Diseases--Popular works. I. Title.
  RC655.B45 2011
  616.4'4--dc23
                                    2011024067

11 12 13 14 15 — 9 8 7 6 5 4 3 2 1
Printed in the United States of America

To my wife, Eileen, who shows me amazing support and who made this happen by believing that I could do this. And to God, who opened doors that no man could have opened. He started this idea in me and showed Himself to be faithful to complete it.

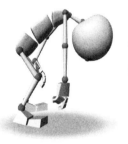

CONTENTS

Foreword by Barbara Wentroble ix

Introduction: Helping You Help Yourself xiii

1 Restorative Care or Symptomatic Relief? 1

2 Stressed? 9

3 A New Approach to Nutrition 25

4 Healthy Eating 33

5 Is Your Thyroid an Underachiever? 59

6 How Much Thyroid Hormone Is Too Much? 85

7 What Hormones and Substances
Inhibit Your Thyroid? 95

8 Tests to Diagnose Thyroid Problems 109

9 Resurrecting the Thyroid 129

10 Struggles With Weight 149

11 The Body Is Always Right 159

Appendix A: Axillary/Basal Temperature Test 167

Appendix B: Artificial Sweeteners. 171

Appendix C: Dr. B's Suggestions. 177

Recommended Thyroid Supplements 177

The A-B-Cs of Calcium 184

Recommended Books About the Thyroid 186

Recommended Websites About the Thyroid........... *187*

Where to Find Nutritionally Oriented Doctors......... *189*

Appendix D: Selected Products That Contain Wheat and
Sources for Alternatives to Wheat 191

Appendix E: "Eating Clean"—Selected Recipes and Tips...... 197

Appendix F: Testimonials................................ 221

Notes 229

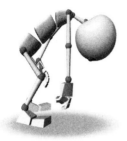

FOREWORD

We are living in the Information Age! People are barraged each day with an overwhelming amount of information through the Internet, satellite TV, phones, and various other types of media. To say that our brains are in overload would be to underestimate the amount of information that reaches our minds each day.

The medical field is no exception when it comes to an enormous amount of information available to the average citizen in the Western world. The challenge is not in needing more information. The problem is in filtering out the unnecessary or bad information from the good and necessary.

Each medical practitioner recommends certain diets or foods to keep you healthy. The problem is that so many of these recommendations are not possible with many people's lifestyle. People who travel are not home to cook certain foods. Some foods are expensive and out of reach for those with limited income. Other foods can be purchased only through the distributor and often taste like cardboard!

Then there are the supplements. By the time you drink enough water to swallow all the recommended supplements each day, there is not any room left for food! That in addition to the high cost of the supplements! Many reports reveal that it is often hard to know if the supplements you buy are actually the quality you need.

Dr. Michael Berglund has done an amazing job in helping us

meet this challenge! He takes the very complex field of preventative medicine and makes it simple to understand. Suggested foods, supplements, healthy recipes, and additional sources of information help the reader to achieve their goals. Dr. Berglund uses a scriptural basis for his recommendations. He even includes symptoms that can determine if you are suffering from thyroid problems. He is the medical friend you have been looking for!

Dr. Berglund's approach to a healthy lifestyle is simple, easy to comprehend, and very doable. Have you ever wanted to sit down and have a doctor talk with you about your thyroid situation in words you could understand? Reading *Tired of Being Sick and Tired* is like sitting down and having a conversation with Dr. Berglund. The reader senses the heart of compassion that is found in this man... the same compassion that was modeled in the life of Jesus.

Readers of this book discover an exciting journey in the life that God planned for His children. His plan was not a life of tiredness and disease. You were created to enjoy an abundant life. Dr. Berglund is like a medical GPS that will help you reach your destination. Read this book, follow the advice given, and enjoy your ride into a healthy future. You deserve this abundant life!

—Barbara Wentroble
Author, Registered Nurse, President of Business Owners for
Christ International

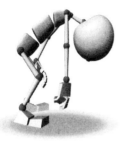

Introduction

HELPING YOU
HELP YOURSELF

Y ou picked up this book because you are looking
for some answers. You want somebody to tell you how to
become healthy. What health issue should you address first? Which
plan should you follow?

You may anticipate that I will inspire and motivate you with my
fantastic teaching and that I will end up putting you on a program
that will change your life, answer all your questions, and help you
achieve all your health goals.

Boy, I hope you're ready to readjust your expectations...I am not
a big "rah-rah" guy. I am not going to whip you into a New Year's
resolution frenzy. That would last only for a short period of time
anyway.

I'm a doctor. But the Latin origin of the word *doctor* is "to teach."
When it comes to helping people become healthy, I see myself first
as a teacher. My job is to help you help yourself. My goal is to undo
all the bad teaching that you've received prior to this, some of which
contradicts the advice I'm about to give you.

I hope to help you improve your instincts. I hope and pray that
the information I provide here will reconnect your mind with your
physical body and show you that you can self-diagnose if you have
the right tools. I want to remove the fear that blocks too many
people from being empowered to improve their own health.

I am a chiropractor, but I did not learn all of this in chiropractic college. I have always had a passion for nutrition and holistic care. In fact, I have been combining it with chiropractic care for at least eighteen of the twenty years I have been in practice. Over those years I have attended three hundred additional hours of postgraduate training, and as I write this, I am about to sit for my board exams, after which I will be certified as a specialist (chiropractic internist), part of the American Board of Chiropractic Internists and the Board of Internal Diagnosis and Disorders.

I am also a Christian. Let me state my conviction emphatically: each of us is uniquely created by God. I hate it when people try to force others to be like they are or try to homogenize us all. The Bible tells us that though we are many, we are one body. (See 1 Corinthians 12:12.) We each have different functions—some do this, some do that—but we need each other.

For instance, the cells that make up the cuticle of your fingernail have no clue how the cells of your liver work. They could argue up and down until they are both red in the face, and they would never see eye to eye on what's important and how best to work out their purpose in the human body. But your cuticle and your liver do not argue. They are glad for each other. They realize that they need each other. This isn't a competition to see who is more important. Your liver doesn't say, "Hey, Cutie, if you're destroyed, I continue to live, but if *I'm* wiped out, this whole body, including you, is a goner." Your liver could say that, but it doesn't.

This comparison works for the human body, for the church, and ultimately for any community, any business, or any organization. All the individual people and parts are made to be different. Each has strengths, but each also has weaknesses.

One-size-fits-all advice never applies to everyone equally. Someone tells you that everyone needs to drink eight 8-ounce glasses of water a day, or drink as many ounces as half their weight in pounds, so if you weigh 200 pounds, you need to drink 100 ounces of water by bedtime. The Mayo Clinic's website issues guidelines about how much fiber you should consume:[1]

❖ Men under age fifty: 38 grams

❖ Men age fifty-one and up: 30 grams

❖ Women under age fifty: 25 grams

❖ Women age fifty-one and up: 21 grams

You can find health rules for everything. Women should have mammograms every year after age fifty. Depending on your age and health history, you should have regular colonoscopies, bone density tests, and stress tests.

Nutritional experts will advise you endlessly, as well. For example:

❖ Calcium and magnesium should always be taken in a 2:1 ratio.

❖ If you're taking fish oil (as the experts say that everyone should), you should take a good antioxidant with it.

❖ Probiotics are very important because if the gastrointestinal system is unhealthy, you can't be healthy.

❖ Vitamin D, believed to be a massively deficient nutrient in America, should be administered in large doses, at least at 2,000 IU a day.

❖ If you're a woman in her childbearing years, you should be taking folic acid.

❖ If you have joint pains, you should be taking glucosamine sulfate, chondroitin sulfates, or MSM to assist with making cartilage so you do not have to be on anti-inflammatory drugs.

❖ Your heart needs CoQ_{10} because heart disease is the number one killer in the United States.

- The website for GNC adds the antioxidants resveratrol (extract from wine) and grape seed extract on their "must-have" list of supplements.[2]

- And if you happen to have a friend who sells supplements (i.e., working for a multilevel marketing company), I'm sure they've come up with other supplements that are "critical" to your health.

You may think I'm going to blast these ideas. I'm not. I'm in favor of them. But everyone doesn't need to take all these supplements. You shouldn't have to take forty pills and supplements every day to be healthy. Your goal in reading books like this, eating well, exercising, and taking supplements should be to reduce your risk factors, to make sure you do not die before your time—not to try to fend off every possible cause of death.

I have a spot on my new patient paperwork that asks people what they are currently taking that is not an over-the-counter or prescription drug (e.g. vitamins, minerals, herbs). Some people write down that they are currently taking more than twenty different supplements. When I ask them why, they say, "That's for my memory. Those two are for my heart. That one is…(pause)…I actually don't remember why I am taking that, but it's supposed to be good for me. I know that. I take this one for…" And the commentary goes on. They've read books, gotten newsletters in the mail, gone online, seen a very compelling infomercial, or maybe even had a nutritional "expert" tell them to start taking this. Now they are seeing me. So obviously some of it didn't work. But there are so many different things, I'm not sure they could tell what's doing what. My response to them is: "Gather a box and load all these supplements in and bring them in on your next visit. We'll go through each one and how much you're taking and determine what is necessary and what I think could be eliminated."

Why do I do that? Because a great number of factors make up your personal health strengths and weaknesses:

+ Your family history

+ Your past injuries

+ Your personality type

+ Your personal health history

+ Your diet

+ Your environment

My family history shows a lot of cardiovascular disease and, to a lesser degree, hypothyroidism. Almost to a person, my relatives have had heart attacks and strokes. Could I develop cancer? Sure. But it's not as likely to happen. I would need to be exposed to some strong environmental causative factors, such as being exposed to radiation or other carcinogens, to kick that up.

My personal blood workup would seem to show that I have trouble with excess carbohydrates. Since cardiovascular disease, an inflammatory issue that is aggravated by carrying extra body weight, an excess intake of carbohydrates, and a deficiency of anti-oxidants, is in my family history, my efforts to stay healthy should focus within this realm. I should keep my diet low in carbohydrates, take antioxidants to minimize any damage from free radicals, and also pay attention to diet and supplementation to make sure that I have lower inflammation levels and less chance of forming clots, which are what cause strokes and blockages in heart disease.

You will find that what I am going to tell you in this book will be refuted by 99 percent of the medical establishment. It is primarily holistic-based care, nutritional at its core. And yet I will tell you to confer with your medical doctor. Why? Because I know it's important to make sure you do not have a tumor in your pituitary gland or active thyroid cancer before starting to follow my advice.

But if you ask your medical doctor what he or she thinks of my nutritional suggestions, you are not likely to hear a resounding confirmation of my advice. Asking many medical doctors about nutrition is the equivalent of asking a handyman how to knit a scarf. The majority of medical doctors have not been trained in nutrition, acupuncture, herbs, or homeopathic health care. Many have never heard of pantethine or policosanol, and they do not know the difference between niacin and niacinamide. These are entirely different paradigms.

Please don't mistake my intentions here. I'm not disparaging medical doctors. They are very smart people who have had a great deal of education. I'm just pointing out that their studies at medical school don't tend to focus on nutrition and holistic treatments.

As we will discuss in the first chapter, the holistic and traditional medical paradigms conflict with each other. The goal is the same: health. But the means for achieving the goal are entirely different. It's like asking a Democrat and Republican how to best achieve a healthy country. The Democrat has one definition of "healthy country," and the Republican has another one, and their opinions are as vastly different as are their modes of getting there.

I can hear your next question: "But who do you think is right?" I will give you a political answer, but I truly believe it. We need both political parties to create balance in our country, and by the same token, we need the differing health paradigms. As much as I believe in my paradigm, I realize that there is a time for a more aggressive approach or more acute life-saving techniques.

My goal in this book is to help *you* to become the expert on *yourself*. I want you to use doctors and websites and books to assist you and to learn how to filter out the bad and allow in the truth. You learn as much as you can, and then you make up your own mind what to do.

Before you start anything, if your loved ones object, tell them that you are not getting better doing what you've been doing, so you are seeking better health through this new protocol. Help them see that you are not satisfied with your health as it stands, and that the medications, doctors, and chiropractors you have consulted have not made enough difference. You just want to be healthier. This new thing might not work either, but then you'll try something else. Help them understand that you are trying to be your own best advocate for your own best health.

At the end of your life, the system you follow will not weep for you if you've been ineffective in your life because of bad health. You will. Authors of books or creators of websites won't stand by you. You will be responsible for what you did in this life.

Blame anybody you want to, but it won't change the fact that you are responsible for taking the best possible care of yourself. Excuses just won't fly: "Well, that surgeon really messed me up." "None of those six weight-loss programs helped me. In fact, after each one, I gained more weight." "My husband never supported me." "I've had a lot of stress to deal with."

I'd rather stand before God and say, "I acknowledge my responsibility for what You gave me to do. I loved You, and I also loved others. You gave me health, and this is what I did with the energy and years you gave me."

Some of you will say, "I can't find a medical doctor to prescribe the thyroid medication that I need." What I hope to provide you in this book is a way around that obstacle. My passion is to help you. How? By removing obstacles and excuses.

I am not a medical doctor, and you are not my patient. I can't take you off your prescriptions. But I can empower you with good health so that you can go into your pharmacy or medical doctor's office to find a way off the medications you are on. Will you be able to stop taking all of them? I don't know. But I do know that once you are on hypertension medications, you will be on them for the rest of your life unless you take steps to change the factors that are causing the increased blood pressure. Same with depression, anxiety, cholesterol, low thyroid, heartburn/reflux, and so forth.[3]

When it comes to your health, the buck stops with you. You're the one who lives in your body. You can figure out if this medication or that supplement is working or is making you sick. If a doctor doesn't acknowledge your side effects on a medication, then you are free to "fire" him or her. If every time I take my car to the mechanic he charges me for stuff that he doesn't fix, I simply won't take my car back there. Granted, I don't understand much about cars, but I do know when somebody doesn't seem to be able to help me.

So my goal for you? It's to help you to help yourself. I hope to set you on a course to make you the world's foremost expert on *you*. You won't have to randomly seek information and experts and blindly follow their programs. Instead, I can teach you to let the Holy Spirit guide you, and the Holy Spirit can help you filter out what's not for you and what is for you. I can't guarantee you success the first time, but since God is putting you on a journey, He will teach you things about yourself through successes and failures.

Remember, according to Jesus's disciple Peter: "His divine power has given us everything we need for life and godliness through our knowledge of him who called us by his own glory and goodness" (2 Pet. 1:3, NIV). I hope that through the information provided in this book, you will be moved forward in your journey with God and you will be able to overcome the health obstacles that have kept you from what He has called you to do.

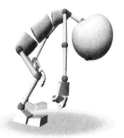

Chapter 1

RESTORATIVE CARE OR SYMPTOMATIC RELIEF?

L et's say you have been diagnosed with gastrointestinal reflux. You may end up taking Zantac, Tagamet, Nexium, Prilosec, or even Prevacid. All of the above drugs turn down or shut off the body's ability to make or secrete stomach acid. At the time of your diagnosis, your health care provider explained the condition and why he or she was prescribing the particular medication. After a short time, you find that the drugs are working well and that your reflux problem has improved or even disappeared. What a relief not to feel the heartburn anymore!

However, no underlying problems have been addressed in the process. Why did you develop the problem in the first place? Will you have to take this drug for the rest of your life? With the symptoms now under control, how will you know what your body was trying to tell you? How will you know if you are well enough to stop taking the medicine? If the problem was brought on by something you did, how will you ever know what to change about your eating habits or your lifestyle?

Your disease did not appear out of nowhere. Red flags should have gone up in your mind when you were handed a prescription without a clear explanation of what you must have done (or not done) to suffer from this condition, not to mention what you should do to fully recover.

What's missing? Restoration.

This is how the medical paradigm works. I like to compare it to putting a strip of black electrical tape over the flashing red oil light on the dashboard of your car and then proclaiming the problem as "fixed." It addresses your symptoms and provides relief from them without paying attention to their underlying causes.

Contrast this with a holistic, restorative approach to health care, in which a person looks at a symptom and says, "This body of mine is trying to tell me about something that is wrong. I need to translate what it's saying and do something about it." In other words, "My car's dashboard oil light is flashing red. It's telling me that the oil in the engine has reached a level that is unhealthy for the engine. I need to add some oil immediately, before additional damage to the engine occurs."

In the holistic model of care, symptoms such as vomiting, diarrhea, a runny nose, excess earwax, swollen tonsils, body odor, and low back spasms are considered to be normal body reactions to negative developments within a person's body. These symptoms cannot be equated with the disease itself, and medicating them away is only a palliative measure.

In holistic terms, diarrhea means that the intestines are trying to rid themselves of something they have deemed harmful, such as a toxin, bad bacteria, or a food to which the person has developed a sensitivity. Doesn't that make sense? Since diarrhea is the body's way of dealing with a problem, the best solution should not be taking a medication to stop the diarrhea. Taking an over-the-counter drug to stop the diarrhea will only keep the irritant in the colon longer, increasing the chance of more damage.

The body is smart. It is trying to prevent disease and heal itself. When the cells of the intestinal lining encounter abnormal bacteria or when toxins enter the gastrointestinal tract, the physical response is, "Remove this as quickly as possible." If this happens early on, vomiting will result. This is a good thing. The body sacrifices comfort in the short term to prevent long-term disease or damage.

By personality, I am nonconfrontational. I dread to hear the words, "Can we talk?" I know they can lead to hours of conversation—oftentimes focused on the fact that I have done something wrong. I prefer peace. However, I have come to realize that the hours of confrontation (if done right) will almost always result in a truer peace, better teamwork, and more contentment. I've come to see that it's worth it. That's another example of enduring short-term pain for the sake of long-term benefit.

A patient came to see me. She had ulcerative colitis, and she had been under the care of a medical doctor. She had received four pints of blood in the previous four weeks because she had lost so much blood via her stools. There really was no hope in sight, which is why she decided to go beyond the medical doctors and specialists and at least "try" me. By her second visit I had determined that she had inflammation in her lower bowels because abnormal bacteria had set up house in her colon, where they were causing excessive inflammation to the point of bleeding. All I needed to do was give her a strong natural antibiotic, and the diarrhea stopped within a week. The bleeding stopped within two weeks. Pretty soon her color returned, and she was back to normal.

To think that she had been suffering for so long with something that was so easily corrected! Unfortunately, this kind of thing happens far too often. This is why I am taking the time to start this book with an in-depth look at the differences between these two paradigms. We need to know what we're dealing with. If the old paradigm we have been relying upon has some major omissions or errors, we need to be able to identify them, admit them, and stop relying on them.

Factoring in More Than Germ Theory

One of the core precepts of the medical paradigm is Louis Pasteur's germ theory. The germ theory, also called the pathogenic theory of medicine, proposes that microorganisms are the cause of many diseases. Although highly controversial when first proposed, it is now a cornerstone of modern medicine and clinical microbiology, leading to such important innovations as antibiotics and better hygienic practices.

Prior to this, people thought that disease was spontaneously generated. Pasteur helped us understand that infectious diseases are spread from one person to the next and that the epidemics and plagues that had devastated populations throughout history up to that point could be prevented or controlled with proper hygiene.

While I agree with this theory, I believe that it should just begin to explain why we become sick. It certainly does not explain why, when one person enters a room with an infectious cough, everyone in the room does not become sick. If there are fifteen people in the room when the sick person coughs, maybe two people will become infected and fall sick, but the other thirteen won't. Why? What factors make the difference? These are factors worth considering.

Hasty Surgical Procedures

The medical paradigm also advocates the surgical removal of "misbehaving" organs. Gallbladders, spleens, ovaries, uteruses, thyroids, tonsils, adenoids, appendixes, and other organs or glands are routinely removed in this country as a first treatment option, without giving any effort to restoring them. Did you know that it is becoming more common for some surgeons to get permission to remove a person's appendix when they are performing abdominal surgery for another reason? The thinking is that people do not need an appendix anyway, and we might as well cut it out before it becomes inflamed (as if to head off a prescheduled rendezvous with appendicitis). And after the removal of glands or organs that are supposed to release hormones into the person's system, medical doctors consider the prescribed synthetic hormones to be just as good as what a healthy person's body can produce on its own.

In contrast, health providers such as me, who follow a holistic model, believe that an organ should be removed only after all other attempts at restoration have been attempted. Surgery remains a viable option, but holistic practitioners will refer to surgeons as a means of last resort, since once an organ has been removed, reversing the situation is all but impossible.

Restoration entails finding out how to help our bodies heal themselves. Notified by various symptoms, we must find all the problems that are associated with the dysfunction in order to restore normal body function. If you start with painkillers, muscle relaxers, anti-inflammatories, or other medications, figuring out the truth (the real problem) really will not be necessary. The chemicals are strong. They will jerry-rig the system to work around the dysfunction. However, with every work-around, one or more new problems may flare up. As in the car-oil analogy above, we are just masking the low-oil warning light by putting black electrical tape over it, thus allowing the engine to be ruined. We won't be aware of the damage until it's irreversible.

Comparing the Holistic and Traditional Models of Medicine

Those who follow the holistic model say:	Those who follow the traditional medical model say:
What's the dysfunction? Where is it?	What's the disease? Name it.
Restoration should always be the first goal.	Substitution is as good as restoration.
Surgery is an option only when all other options have been tried or for emergency situations.	Surgery is a viable first option for nonvital organs and glands.

Those who follow the holistic model say:	Those who follow the traditional medical model say:
We should not ask, "What can we remove and still survive?" Our bodies will work best with all of their organs functioning at optimum levels. Living well is always better than living long.	What can we survive without? Saving lives is the priority, even if it means living at a lower level of function.
Symptoms are the body talking to us about the underlying problem.	Masking symptoms = fixing the problem.
The body is very smart.	Our bodies have no real intrinsic ability to heal themselves, and they are not very smart. Our bodies need a qualified expert to do the work of thinking for them.
The parts of the body are connected. A problem in one part can create secondary issues in an entirely different part of the body.	The body is a system of compartments. "Which specialist do I need to send you to?"
The body knows how to do things better than we might think it does. If we remove obstacles and provide for its needs, we can expect the body to heal itself.	Help comes from outside. "You can't do the work. Let me do it for you."

New Testament Parallels

Interestingly, the holistic approach to health care parallels the biblical view of the body of people known as the church. This well-known passage of New Testament Scripture compares the church to a human body:

> For even as the body is one and yet has many members, and all the members of the body, though they are many, are one body, so also is Christ....For the body is not one member, but many. If the foot says, "Because I am not a hand, I am not a part of the body," it is not for this reason any the less a part of the

body. And if the ear says, "Because I am not an eye, I am not a part of the body," it is not for this reason any the less a part of the body. If the whole body were an eye, where would the hearing be? If the whole were hearing, where would the sense of smell be? But now God has placed the members, each one of them, in the body, just as He desired. If they were all one member, where would the body be? But now there are many members, but one body. And the eye cannot say to the hand, "I have no need of you"; or again the head to the feet, "I have no need of you." On the contrary, it is much truer that the members of the body which seem to be weaker are necessary; and those members of the body which we deem less honorable, on these we bestow more abundant honor.... But God has so composed the body... so that there may be no division in the body, but that the members may have the same care for one another. And if one member suffers, all the members suffer with it; if one member is honored, all the members rejoice with it.

—1 CORINTHIANS 12:12–26

Within the local church, if one of the members struggles with something, acting dysfunctionally, how does God want us to respond? As we can see from the abundant advice in the New Testament, He wants us to figure out the problem and correct it. If someone has become alienated, He wants us to make every effort to lovingly restore that person to a right relationship with God and with his or her local church family.

How can we figure out the problem? We watch that person, and we talk to him or her. We pray. We look for the truth. There is a reason when somebody acts up or sins. There is a reason when people do not fit in or refuse to participate with others in the body of Christ.

If I have a pain in my knee, the easy solution would be to take ibuprofen or some kind of painkiller. Poof. The pain is gone. But the dysfunction remains. If I have "issues" and I act like a creep around women, my church could attempt to solve the problem by simply barring me from women-oriented ministries and asking someone to keep an eye on me. But that won't heal my problem, will it? Instead, I need their help to figure out what started this, why I continue in this pattern, and what I can do to change it. I need to have God and His people come alongside me to help me clean up the mess and become a new creature. Sure, managing my "creepiness" is easier and less time-consuming, but we can all agree that I won't be healed or restored as a result.

In other words, God's way of attaining healthy "body life" is *restoration*, even if it requires extreme patience and much wisdom. He does not want us to numb the pain or banish the troublemaker.

My approach to health care is like that, holistic and restorative. I will use Band-Aids when I must, but I prefer to keep a symptom in plain view so I can determine if my solution is working.

That is why, in this book about solutions to thyroid problems, I will discuss so many different symptomatic road markers—along with an equal number of commonsense approaches to lovingly healing and restoring health and integration to your entire body.

Your body has been "wonderfully made" (Ps. 139:14). I want you to grow in your awe and respect for that fact as you come to explore its intricacies with me in the following chapters.

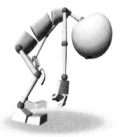

Chapter 2

STRESSED?

All of us live with dysfunction. Most of the time, as our bodies are trying to handle it, they will let us know if we should change something. The way our bodies "speak up" is through physical and emotional symptoms.

I like to think of symptoms as your body's version of your car's warning lights. I find it somewhat funny that people call these warning lights "idiot lights." Even as I am writing this chapter, my dashboard happens to be showing a yellow picture of a car part with the word "CHECK" inside it. The problem is—I don't know what the heck this part is. I'm not a car person. I do not know what the parts look like. So I don't know if what they are showing me is an engine or an alternator. *What* should I check? It doesn't really matter because I'm going to take it to the mechanic tomorrow so he can hook it up to his computer and diagnose the problem. Those idiot lights make me feel like an idiot, all right.

My car story exemplifies how many people feel about their bodies. Perhaps you are one of them. You are with you all day long, and yet you do not understand what your symptoms mean. You develop a headache. Why? The delightful commercials tell you it's not important to know why; you just need to take two Excedrins (which, by the way, is a combination of aspirin and the same amount of caffeine as one cup of coffee or two cans of Mountain Dew[1]). No one suggests to you that your body may actually be trying to communicate with you.

I have mastered Spanish up to the high school level and no further. My language ability is barely sufficient for communicating to Spanish-speaking people. I certainly cannot serve as a translator from Spanish to English. However, I have become proficient at interpreting the language of the human body. I have been training for years to learn how to translate symptoms to patients so they can know what their bodies' "idiot lights" are telling them.

If you can't figure out what your physical symptoms are telling you, do not waste time feeling stupid. My first few weeks of Spanish class included me saying *hola* and *adios* and—many times—*no comprendo*, "I don't understand." My teacher didn't make me feel stupid. She believed that eventually I would be able to carry on a conversation with someone in Spanish.

In a similar way, you are only beginning to improve your ability to analyze what your body is saying. When a symptom starts bothering you, just say, "I need to take it to the expert (doctor) to have him 'hook me up to the computer.'" If you visit a holistic physician like me, your office visit can be part of your education process. Holistic health care providers can be your language instructors. If you do not have anyone in your area, my hope is that this book will inspire you to want to learn to communicate with your body. You'll start slowly. However, with experience, you too can learn what your body is trying to tell you.

Learning the Language

Back in the 1990s I used a computer software company that had the ability to log on to my machine remotely to fix problems. When I couldn't figure out what was keeping my software from loading up properly or otherwise not running as it was supposed to, they used this software called "pcAnywhere" to call up my computer via the modem. Then they would be in control of my computer. I would watch them as they figured out the problem I was having. It was weird watching the technicians control my screen from twenty-two hundred miles away.

Since I am fairly cheap inherently, I would watch them closely to see how they fixed things. What did they do? What did they enter? How did they fix the problem? After seeing them in action a couple of times, I stopped calling the customer support (which charged me for each tech support call), because now I could solve this problem just as easily as they could. Eventually I figured out what I had been doing in the first place to create the problem. Pretty soon I didn't have that problem anymore.

The truth is that most of our problems require people with more expertise than we possess. Yet at the same time, you and I can learn from the experts. Situations such as the one above can build your confidence that you can, with practice, understand things that used to be beyond your comprehension. In particular, you can learn what your body is telling you and how to handle a recurring health situation.

Naturally, it will take some experimentation and patience on your part, but eventually you'll develop it. The first few times the solution may go against what doctors have told you and maybe even against your own logic. I have had several patients with bad cases of reflux and heartburn. When I told them to supplement with extra stomach acid, it seemed counterintuitive to them. You should have seen their disbelieving faces when I told them what I wanted them to do. I reassured them, "Look, take one pill with your meal, and if it develops worse, you can take some baking soda to neutralize the acid. But if the reflux feels better, then keep increasing your acid dose until you are without symptoms." And it worked for them.

Stress: Can't Live With It,
Can't Live Without It

I could (and hope to do this in the future) write a whole book on stress. A heightened stress level aggravates health issues and makes you take notice of them.

Stress is all around. You may feel you have a lot of stress in your life, but what you really have are *stressors*. Stressors are external factors. Stress is how you let those stressors affect you.

Yes. I did say how you *let* them affect you. You can have some control.

If you tell me that your stress is far above and beyond other people's stress, surely I can find someone with more. I have patients whose kids are heroin addicts and whose parents are on their deathbeds. I know parents whose adult children were in motor vehicle accidents that caused brain damage, and they are now taking care of them for the rest of their lives. I know a wife whose husband is addicted to crack and who, to support his addiction, keeps stealing from her.

You do not need an excuse to blame for your stress; you need to learn to identify the stressors so you can manage or even overcome them. You are an overcomer. What is standing in opposition to what you want or need to do right now? That's a stressor, and it's also an obstacle. The question is, how will you overcome the obstacles?

The Bible speaks about being refined by fire. Want to know something? The only way to grow involves going through adversity. Both self-imposed challenges and outside situations become your opportunities to mature and grow strong as you draw closer to God. To be an overcomer and to grow stronger, you need to go through the fire (not letting it stop you and certainly not expecting to be instantaneously transported past it), and you need to know that God is with you each step of the way.

One of my patients was having difficulty sleeping, and she had a rapid heart rate. I evaluated her. I felt that the problem wasn't her heart. It wasn't excessive hormones. It was anxiety. We started talking about what was going on. She was having a hard time with how someone had treated her. She felt cheated and swindled. This situation was the source of her anxiety. I talked with her about how to approach it. We had already decided not to medicate it, but should she fight against it (had Satan brought on this situation to prevent her from doing what God wanted her to do?)—or could she recognize the hand of God in this? Was He allowing her to reap what she had sown in order to teach her something? Could she now turn to Him in her weakness, thus becoming stronger than before? Could she trust in His full control over her life?

Being depressed, anxious, and worried are not effective ways of dealing with stressors; they are only symptoms of the underlying problems. In her case I prayerfully advised her to seek God's peace and total faith in His control to set the situation right again, trusting that His way is best.

We weren't meant to worry or be anxious. Did you know that? God created human beings to walk with Him in the Garden of Eden; in other words, to be in perfect relationship with Him and to look to Him to supply all our needs. The situation with the forbidden fruit changed that. After that, the relationship with God became strained. A wall went up between people and God. Stressors became the norm.

Then Jesus came to take down the wall. He came so that our relationship with God could be restored, so that the Holy Spirit could indwell us, comfort us, and help us. Our challenge now is to learn to live in His peace all the time, to not let anyone steal our joy, to praise God in every situation, to rely on His power to deliver us out of trouble, and, above all, not to rely on ourselves.

Even when He allows us to remain in less than pleasant situations, He is still working. Nothing catches Him off guard. He always hears our prayers, and He is always in control. Do we trust Him? Or do we revert to trusting in our own methods?

When we trust in our own strength, the inevitable result is anxiety or worry. More than three hundred times the Bible tells us to stay away from worry and fear. Look up some of these passages about worry and fear (key words are based on the New American Standard version of the Bible) to see how clear the message is:

"Do Not Be Afraid"

Genesis 43:23; 46:3; 50:19, 21; Exodus 20:20; Deuteronomy 20:1, 3; 31:6; Joshua 11:6; Judges 4:18; 1 Samuel 4:20; 22:23; 23:17; 28:13; 2 Kings 1:15; 19:6; 25:24; Nehemiah 4:14; Psalm 49:16; Proverbs 3:25; Isaiah 37:6; 44:8; Jeremiah 1:8; 40:9; 42:11 (twice); Ezekiel 3:9; Daniel 10:12, 19; Zephaniah 3:16; Matthew 1:20; 14:27; 17:7; 28:5, 10; Mark 5:36; 6:50; Luke 1:13, 30; 2:10; 8:50; 12:4, 32; John 6:20; Acts 18:9; 27:24; Revelation 1:17

"Do Not Fear"

Genesis 15:1; 21:17; 26:24; 35:17; Exodus 14:13; Numbers 14:9; 21:34; Deuteronomy 1:21, 29; 3:2, 22; 31:8; Joshua 8:1; 10:8, 25; Judges 6:10 ("...you shall not fear the gods of the Amorites..."), 23; Ruth 3:11; 1 Samuel 12:20; 2 Samuel 9:7; 13:28; 1 Kings 17:13; 2 Kings 6:16; 17:35, 37–38 ("You shall not fear other gods..."); 1 Chronicles 22:13; 28:20; 2 Chronicles 20:15, 17; 32:7; Job 21:9 ("Their houses are safe from fear"); Psalms 64:4; 78:53 ("He led them safely, so that they did not fear"); Isaiah 7:4 ("...have no fear..."); 10:24; 35:4 ("...fear not"); 40:9; 41:10, 13–14; 43:1, 5; 44:2; 51:7; 54:4 ("Fear not"), 14 ("You will be far from oppression, for you will not fear"); Jeremiah 10:5; 30:10 ("Fear not"); 46:27–28; Lamentations 3:57; Joel 2:21–22; Haggai 2:5; Zechariah 8:13, 15; Matthew 10:26, 28, 31; Luke 5:10; 12:7; John 12:15 ("Fear not"); 14:27 ("Do not let your heart be troubled, nor let it be fearful."); 1 Peter 3:14; Revelation 2:10

"Do Not Be Troubled"

John 14:1 ("Do not let your heart be troubled..."); Acts 20:10

"Fearful"

Matthew 8:26, KJV ("Why are ye fearful, O ye of little faith?"); Mark 4:40, KJV ("Why are ye so fearful?"); Revelation 21:8, KJV ("But the fearful...shall have their part in the lake which burneth with fire and brimstone...")

Naturally, despite all of this advice and even these biblical warnings, people still worry themselves sick. Most of us think it's normal.

Now I realize that there's a very large gray zone between someone who is a totally worry-filled, freaked-out spaz and a person who is at peace, utterly trusting God. People in the gray zone tend to use alternative terms such as, "I'm just concerned." How concerned are you? Is your concern keeping you up at night? Are you, in fact, pretty anxious?

Of course, I may not be the best judge of anxiety levels, because I am way too laid-back. That means that much of my peace does not really come from a place of trust but rather from eternal optimism—with a side helping of lazy. I don't worry very much. Things usually work out for me. I never turn molehills into mountains. In fact, a lot of the time I reduce my very real mountains into little molehills. Sometimes, my wife needs to point this out: "Why didn't you see that this was a problem?" Obviously, I downgraded it on the problem scale.

Some of you are planners. You control your anxiety by controlling your situations. You do not worry because you have installed safety nets underneath your safety nets five levels deep in case the one above it fails.

But whether you plan away your anxiety, you're as laid-back as I am, or you're somewhere in between, it's likely that you need some help in your battle against stress. As you learn how to read your personal "anxiety meter," you can also learn how to put your complete trust in God, day by day and situation by situation.

Worrying Ourselves Sick

Stress weakens us. Whenever researchers have put animals in stressful situations or have taken a look at prisoners who have undergone extensive torture, the result has been the same: under stress, their bodily systems have aged. Their muscles and ligaments have grown weaker. Their bones have become more fragile. Their brains begin to atrophy. Their immune systems have gone haywire.

The adrenal glands serve as the main stress glands of your body. They are small glands, weighing only about five grams each, located on the top of each kidney. They release epinephrine (adrenaline), norepinephrine (noradrenaline), cortisol, aldosterone, and DHEA. You need them all.

(Did you know that caffeine grabs some of the adrenaline that your body is storing for emergency rations and uses it for today? That's the equivalent of paying your rent or mortgage with a credit card. Bad idea.)

Your body has two modes it functions in: *sympathetic* and *parasympathetic*.

The parasympathetic mode maintains your body. In this mode your organs work well, food is digested, and tissues are repaired. The body works, while it also rests, much like a town in which the roads are repaved, the potholes are filled, the grass is mowed, and streets are cleaned. It's business as usual.

In the town analogy, "sympathetic mode" is not business as usual. It means that the town is in a state of emergency. A tornado has been spotted just west of town. A flood threatens to engulf the area. A blizzard has caused all the roads to be impassable. The power plant is down. Aliens are landing in the Walmart parking lot. (Just wondering if you're paying attention here.)

All of these situations force the townspeople to discontinue normal operations and shift employees into emergency activities. Nobody's going to worry about mowing grass or filling potholes if half the town is under water. In fact, we may even need to call in the National Guard to help us function.

As far as your body is concerned, when your body shifts away from normal functions such as digestion and repair, it declares a state of emergency. Adrenaline sounds the alarm. Sympathetic mode and stress mode are the same thing.

You may have heard the phrase "fright, fight, or flight." This refers to stress mode or survival mode. A fear-inducing incident occurs, and suddenly it's life or death, do or die. You are being chased by a mountain lion. Your child has fallen off a cliff and is hanging from a branch eight feet down. Someone is holding a gun to your head.

What happens in this sympathetic mode? In one word: adrenaline. Your body releases adrenaline. This causes a priority shift within your body. No longer does it concern itself with digestion or good bowel function. (In fact, you may lose control of either one.) Your body will not spend any effort or time on healing or repair or building strong bones. Blood purification via liver detoxification moves way down on the list.

In sympathetic mode, the last thing your body wants to do is give you pain signals to warn you what not to do. This is the time when someone with broken leg manages to crawl out of his car a minute before the car explodes.

With normal functions deprioritized, what does your body focus on? It focuses on increasing blood supply to your brain to insure clear decision making via increased blood pressure, along with increased heart rate and stroke volume (the amount of blood squeezed by each contraction). Your arteries shunt the blood from your organs to your the muscles of your arms and legs so that you will be ready for running ("flight") or exercising increased strength ("fight"). Your blood sugar increases as fuel for your cells. Whatever it takes to survive a threat, your body stands poised for action: think quick, move quick, be strong, survive, or help someone else survive.

Sounds like a great mechanism, right? Absolutely. We have a great Architect. However, the problem is that we have lost track of what is truly life threatening. Our distant ancestors needed to defend themselves against serious, imminent stressors—warmongering invaders, starvation, wild animals, and more. We really don't have too many of those life-threatening hazards in modern-day society. For us, our sympathetic mode kicks in as a result of chronic stress. Our warmongering invader may be our depleted checkbook. Our wild animal might be the recent rumors of a corporate downsizing.

As life piles up and starts to seem out of control, our "fright, fight, or flight" mechanism ends up working overtime.

Many of our stressors are beyond our control: the loss of a job, the death of a loved one, chronic pain, financial hardship, marriage issues. But we can learn how to limit our stress responses, to "dial down" and to enjoy better health as a result.

How to Tell If You're Stressed

You were not wired to live in a state of chronic stress. Look what happens when you feel stressed. Because your body has decided that certain things are not important, you no longer make acid in your stomach, which sets you up for malabsorption and an increased chance for ulcers and gastritis. Since a full-functioning immune system does not help you when you're being chased by a lion, infections can develop a foothold.

If you find that hard to believe, think back to the last time you carried the responsibility for a major project or event. You were carrying a heavy stress load, and a lot of people were relying on you. You weren't sure you would be able to complete it, but then you did. There were a few fires that needed to be put out, but you did it. Then the next day or the day after that, you got sick or you slept for a day. That's adrenal burnout. You didn't ask your sympathetic system to kick in, but it responded subconsciously. It enabled you to stay up until late at night in order to get the job done. As far as your body could tell subconsciously, this was a life-and-death situation.

Why did you become sick? Because your body had pushed and pushed, suppressing all signals or warnings, until the job was done. Then, in order to replenish in parasympathetic mode, you had to be knocked down. Metaphorically, I like to describe the adrenal glands as a bucket, reserved for emergencies. If you use it up, you need to provide for a time of replenishment. Your adrenal system cannot be considered a bottomless well of supply. It can run dry. When this happens, it's called adrenal fatigue.

Symptoms of Adrenal Fatigue

Adrenal fatigue, sometimes to the point of adrenal exhaustion, occurs either as a result of having an already weak stress system or by overdoing it. People with a weak stress/adrenal system have very distinct symptoms, which I've summarized below:

+ **Low blood pressure.** People who have had lifelong problems dealing with adrenal fatigue will note, "My blood pressure has always been low." They say it with a sense of pride, and although I realize that they do not have the risk factors associated with high blood pressure, they will have a number of problems associated with adrenal weakness.

+ **"Head rush."** When people with low blood pressure stand up too quickly, they can experience a sensation of near-fainting, odd sensations in their heads, or blacked-out vision.

+ **Ciliary muscle endurance.** The brighter the light, the smaller the pupil of a person's eye should become in order to protect the retina and allow the person to see in different light levels. The ciliary muscles of persons with adrenal fatigue will initially constrict but then eventually pulsate between bigger and smaller or just open back up again despite the fact that the bright light is still shining in their eyes.

+ **Moodiness.** People who have adrenal fatigue will seem fine one moment only to break into tears or an angry tirade the next moment, for almost no reason. For people whose emotions are more hidden, this may take the form of being "easily frustrated" or "short" with others.

+ **Hypersensitive senses.** An individual with adrenal fatigue may need to wear sunglasses outside (and maybe even inside in a bright room). This will be the first person in a room to complain of how loud the radio or television is, and this person will also tend to complain about a lady's overpowering perfume two tables over at a restaurant.

In other words, the five senses of a person with adrenal fatigue have a small "acceptability window."

* **Susceptibility to viral infections.** Since healthy adrenal function in the body provides a safety net under the immune system, I have found that adrenal fatigue seems to make a person prone to catch colds, the flu, and other viral infections like mononucleosis, herpes (oral and genital), papilloma viruses (warts), chicken pox, and many more.

* **Low blood sugar.** Individuals with adrenal fatigue are prone to plummeting blood sugar if they miss a meal.

* **Intake of sugar or carbohydrates.** Persons with adrenal fatigue self-medicate with sugar, carbohydrates, or caffeine in order to feel better. Waking up can be a struggle for these individuals. Typically not "morning people," they may also want to take a nap in the middle of the afternoon between 1:00 and 4:00 p.m.

Cortisol Too

Guess what? The worst part is not only the adrenaline secreted when the person goes into sympathetic mode. It is also how the adrenal glands release cortisol in addition to the adrenaline—and cortisol acts to suppress the function of the thyroid gland. This represents an intentional conservation of physical energy, again because it doesn't make sense to waste the body's energy with repair and replacement of tissues when a lion is chasing you. But when we're talking about chronic stress, it becomes a problem.

Supplements (pills and creams) can help pull cortisol out of a person's system. However, I prefer to see people not become hypersecreters of adrenaline and cortisol in the first place.

Eating properly helps your body to repair itself and to remain in a less-stressed condition. For starters, I recommend less or even no caffeine, no refined sugar or high-fructose corn syrup, and no white flour (processed from wheat). See the next chapter for additional information about nutrition.

Also, find out about possible food sensitivities, and avoid those food items. Many people find that, in addition to the refined carbohydrates mentioned above, they cannot tolerate dairy products (especially pasteurized ones) and many different grains.

Good and Bad Responses to Stressors

In addition to all the wonderful promises of God, Jesus promises us that in this life we will have troubles. (See John 16:33.) He didn't say "maybe" or "it's possible," but "you will." The Bible reminds us that we cannot avoid persecution and being refined by fire. It also promises that joy will follow the tears. In the midst of our troubles, we need to believe that God is in control.

David started many of his psalms lamenting about how ticked he was, how life wasn't fair, how the persecution was too much, or how the ungodly people were getting what they didn't deserve. Invariably, by the end of the psalm (in other words, by the end of his prayer), he would be saying "But You are God" or "You are just" or "In You I trust."

The Bible tells us that David was "a man after God's heart" (1 Sam. 13:14; Acts 13:22), and we need to have hearts like that. We need to pray in order to be on God's page. Otherwise we cannot figure out if some stressor is coming from heaven or from hell. Sometimes when the source of our stress turns out to be the adversary, we need to use our authority in Christ to send it packing.

Do you have a hard time identifying good versus bad and helpful versus harmful? Let me clue you in. Bad stress is loaded with fear—fear of rejection, fear of losing someone or something (job, house, credit rating), fear of pain, fear of death, and more. Negative emotions fuel this type of stress.

God Doesn't Want Us to Be Stressed

The last thing in the world God wants His children to be is stressed. He made us to walk with Him in a perfect relationship of trust and dependence. We develop stress because we do not have that close Eden-like relationship with Him we are supposed to have. Because we do not know God very well, we fail to understand His nature and how much He loves us and wants the best for us; therefore we do not trust Him.

We fear unknown outcomes. When we want to avoid one or more possible outcomes to a difficult situation, we decide to take matters into our own hands. Of course, that usually means worrying over stuff over which we have no real control, but at least we feel that someone is paying attention to the problem. Somehow we interpret insomnia or wringing our hands with anxiety as effective against the fearful outcomes we are facing.

I tell people that our part in the equation should involve controlling our actions because God controls the results. When you are stressed, remember this 1-2-3 response:

1. "God, is this from You?"

2. "God, what do You want me to do in this situation?"

3. Then let God work.

If some stressor keeps trying to push its way into your worry center, just keep saying, "God, I trust You." Do not be afraid to ask Him for help to trust Him more. So what if one way He will build your faith involves facing more difficulties? Remember the scripture, "Better is one day in your courts than a thousand elsewhere" (Ps. 84:10, NIV). Better is poverty with God than riches without. Better is sickness with a close relationship with God than good health and no relationship.

In Luke 11:9–10 we read, "So I say to you, ask, and it will be given to you; seek, and you will find; knock, and it will be opened to you.

For everyone who asks, receives; and he who seeks, finds; and to him who knocks, it will be opened." The form of these Greek verbs implies persistent action—"ask and keep on asking"; "seek and keep on seeking"; "knock and keep on knocking." I might add, "Relate and keep on relating to God." We need to overcome our sense of futility and keep on keeping on. God truly is the source of peace for us.

To be sure, we need to find out if what we keep asking for is God's will. We need to figure out if our prayers represent our own idea of the best solution to a problem, or if we desire the fullness of heavenly provision. Jesus's words spoken in Gethsemane should come out of our mouths: "Yet not My will, but Yours be done" (Luke 22:42). Paul prayed three times for a "thorn" from Satan to be removed from him, and God denied his request, telling him that in his weakness, Paul would become strong (2 Cor. 12:7–10).

I realize that I'm giving you pie-in-the-sky advice. "In a perfect world, dot dot dot," right? How does this really work? How can you *not* let your circumstances determine your mood or affect your peace? Sometimes you can enter a room feeling chipper, but as soon as you talk to someone, read an e-mail or a text message, or even watch the news on TV, you're anxious, annoyed, or just plain angry.

The fact of the matter is that your battle is not against flesh and blood (your boss, your spouse, or even your noisy neighbors). Your battle is against your human tendency to pin the blame on someone or something—and then to wrestle with it yourself. You really can turn your anxious struggles over to God. It may take a significant amount of practice to make this your "default" response to difficulties, but He will help you to trust Him.

Once you develop a taste of that "peace of God, which transcends all understanding" (Phil. 4:7, NIV), you will know that nothing else matters and that God is truly in control. Your whole life needs to be about keeping that peace. It's part of the fruit of the Spirit ("love, joy, peace, patience, kindness, goodness, faithfulness, gentleness, self-control…" Gal. 5:22–23). That peace furnishes internal evidence that you are believing God and in a right relationship with Him.

The opposite of peace is anxiety. Anxiety is another word for fear. It's not a disease per se, although it can be a symptom of physical problems. Anxiety can also be a spiritual state, and it certainly responds to the loving, capable Spirit of God.

I believe that we can "pray off" fear like an unwelcome entity. When the Bible says that God gave you "a spirit not of fear but of power and love and self-control" (2 Tim. 1:7, ESV), the words imply that fear can be a spirit. By yourself or with the help of a friend, try casting off a specific fear—give it a name, such as fear of sickness—and state aloud your trust in God. Claim peace and joy because of your position of trust. Take hold of the fear that something bad will happen, admitting honestly that it could happen but acknowledging to God that you are willing to go through it if He wants you to. Ask Him to help you not only overcome the fear but also grow from overcoming it. Ask Him to make you into a testimony to His character and power.

If your stressor is an unpleasant individual, make it a point to respond with kindness. Try not to participate in complaining sessions with others. You do not have to be a doormat, but if you need to stand up for yourself, make sure that you go in there filled with God's peace so your own emotions do not have a chance to take over.

Jesus tells you, "Come to me, all you who are weary and burdened, and I will give you rest. Take my yoke upon you and learn from me, for I am gentle and humble in heart, and you will find rest for your souls. For my yoke is easy and my burden is light" (Matt. 11:28–30, NIV).

I know. Some of you just need rest. All God asks is that you come to *Him* for it. It's easy to do that. Don't make it too complicated.

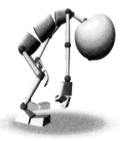

Chapter 3

A NEW APPROACH TO NUTRITION

Before you start reading this chapter, I want you to raise your right hand. Go ahead. Do it. You can hold the book with your left hand. Raise your right hand and repeat the following:

> I, [state your name], do solemnly swear that I will not become a food Nazi and judge others by their food choices (especially after reading this chapter). I realize that what might be good for my family or for me is not necessarily what others need to do. I refuse to judge others. I realize that as soon as I start judging, someone else who is even more restrictive with food choices will judge my food choices and me. This book is a tool for me to develop healthy eating habits. I may feel led to help others eat better, but I will not use the information that I read here to pummel people into submission.

OK, now that we have that out of the way, let me tell you a story. My wife, Eileen, was at church on a Wednesday to teach a class to the middle schoolers. She got there early, so she went to the vending machine to buy a bottle of water. Unfortunately, once she put her money in there and pushed the "water" button, the machine flashed a message that the vending machine had no water bottles left. The rest of my wife's choices were all sodas. She was thirsty, so she chose an orange soda. She proceeded back to the middle school room where the regular instructor (we'll call this woman Doris) was. As soon as Doris saw Eileen, she commented, "You're drinking that?"

Eileen was confused. "What do you mean?"

Doris repeated, "Well, I can't believe that you're drinking…*that.*" (This was stated as though Eileen had taken a glass and scooped water right out of the toilet and was about ready to put the glass up to her lips.) Evidently this woman knew that Eileen was also a chiropractor who taught people the benefits of healthy eating and drinking.

Doris had decided to hold Eileen to a food and drink standard that our family does not participate in. This happens to us a lot. People see us at a fast-food drive-through, and they comment (with that same toilet-water look), "I thought you guys were vegetarians or something." Nope.

The truth is this: we have not made rigid food rules in our home. We understand about making food choices that contribute to a healthy lifestyle. We are not trying to impress anyone. Now when people look disappointed at us, unable to figure out how we could stoop so low, we just look at each other and say, "It's just orange soda…"

While you may need to make perfect dietary choices until your body recovers from ailments and prior abuse, and you do need to figure out which foods were making you sick and which ones are good for you, you do not need to be so strict with yourself forever. I tell my patients initially (right after which they say, "In moderation, right?") that they have to be nearly perfect up front so their bodies can heal. But I hope that all of this work now will free them up so that in the future they feel free to go to someone's home and eat whatever gets put in front of them or even order a pizza sometimes.

No More Rules

If you pick up this book and expect me to give you all the rules to follow in order to become healthy, you will probably be disappointed.

Jesus rebuked the Pharisees, who "tie up heavy burdens and lay them on men's shoulders, but they themselves are unwilling to move them with so much as a finger" (Matt. 23:4). I have written this book to help you become healthy, not to burden you. I want to help you take your life back. I want to help you *not* to spend so much money, time, and effort going to doctors. I realize that when you are tired and chronically ill or in pain, you spend an inordinate amount of time focusing on yourself and your own needs. I do not believe that we've been put here on Earth in order to be introspective and self-focused. Instead I believe that we need to spend only enough time on ourselves to make us able to go out and effectively do the work that God has put in front of us.

Think of it this way. If I showed you a jalopy of a car, most of you would be unimpressed. You'd see a rusty, unusable car that is way past its prime and that needs to be junked. But someone else could walk up to that hunk of junk and see the potential in it. They could see that this is a 1966 Mustang Shelby GT350, and they would know that they could rebuild it back to original condition. Wow! (Don't be too impressed. I'm not a car guy. I had to look up online what might be a great collector car.)

When I see people living in dysfunction, my first idea is not to just jerry-rig them to keep them functioning, I want to restore them back as close to factory original as possible. Many of you are probably saying, "Your point is...?" Here is why I'm giving you this comparison. Some of you may feel like that car. I'm telling you that once you get your car (body) back to functioning fabulously, you will not need to spend two hours a day waxing and wiping it down and applying conditioner to the leather interior to keep it in mint condition. You won't be afraid to invite passengers, lest they stain or damage the interior. You won't be afraid to drive it because it could get dinged. The purpose of restoring a car is not to have a trophy car. The purpose is to drive it and use it.

I had a roommate once named Pete, and he had a red Volkswagen GTI. To me, this car was just a souped-up version of the VW Golf, a hatchback compact car—a nice one, but still just a hatchback. He had friends with far sportier and more expensive imports, but I guarantee that they didn't take better care of their car than Pete did. He was out there on Saturdays waxing and cleaning that car. He made sure that car had the best sound system that money could buy. And he would brag that he got it up to 110 miles an hour on a remote highway. Again, you'd think he had a Ferrari. Pete took good care of that car's insides and outsides—and he used it daily.

I want to help you take good care of your body. I do not want you to become obsessive, but I want you to be a bit more protective and nurturing than you probably have been in the past. Your body will not necessarily keep working well no matter what you throw into it. If I try to use vegetable oil in my car's engine instead of motor oil, saying, "Oil is oil," you would think I was an idiot.

I might insist, "Well, when I put it in, it started right up and ran just fine."

You'd retort, "Sure, it runs well for the moment. But if you keep trying to run your engine with cooking oil in it, you will do long-term damage to your car." And although I'm not a car guy, I think you'd be right. The car was made to function with a certain type of oil, oil of a certain viscosity.

In the same way, your body was made with specific needs. Just because you see people smoking two packs of cigarettes a day and living until they are eighty years old doesn't mean that smoking isn't bad for them. Their longevity represents a testimony to the Maker of their body, not to whether or not smoking abuses the human body.

The same One who created us created the plants and animals we share the earth with. We were made for them, and they were made for us. The more we change what the Creator made or try to be a creator, devising replacement foods, the more chronic, degenerative disease we're going to notice. Sure, like the car, the engine will run awhile on vegetable oil, but eventually, the wear and tear in the cylinders will show up. The heat from the friction will warp the rings and the engine will no longer be powerful. Instead, it will be able to accelerate only very slowly—and eventually not at all. Do you feel something like that starting to happen to you?

Look. My goal is not to make you uptight about food, water, chemicals, toxins, pesticides, and anything else you can think of. If I do that, I will have robbed you of your peace, which will guarantee that you *won't* be healthy. That's a fact.

I have read many natural health care books. As far as I'm concerned, most of them go too far. They are way too rigid and bound by rules. I do not want this one to be like that.

Rule-Free Living

Let me repeat: I hate rules. I hate rules because even good rules are so impossible to follow. When keeping the Old Testament rules turned out to be unachievable, God was finally able to show people the futility of attempting to follow rules in order to be good enough. Rules and laws do not save people. God saves people. He sent His Son Jesus to fulfill the collection of rules called the Law, so that forevermore people could be good enough for the kingdom of God by means of faith in Him. The name Jesus comes from two simple words put together: "Jehovah saves."

The Greek word *sozo* is translated in the New American Standard Bible into "save," "saved," "saves," and "saving." Depending on its context, the word is also translated as "to bring safely," "cured," "to ensure salvation," "to get well," "made well," "preserved," "recover," and "restore." To call Him "Jehovah saves" means that Jesus is the Savior—and that Jesus heals.

Rules do not save or heal. I watch the television show *The Biggest Loser* on which massively overweight individuals vie for the title of biggest loser. Typical winners of the show lose two hundred pounds or more over an eight-month period, which is usually more than 50 percent of their body weight. What does it take for these people to lose seven to twenty pounds a week for that long? It requires five or six hours a day in the gym and the rest of the time preparing food and doing weigh-ins and challenges. The system does work. *The Ultimate Workout* is a spinoff product that enables people to undertake the system at home. However, I don't have time to be Bob and Jillian with my patients, nor do they have time (or the money) to hire a trainer and work out that much.

I believe that many health books are asking you to perform the equivalent of spending six hours a day in the gym. They give you every dietary/nutritional piece of advice ever discovered and simply say, "Just follow all of them. Be perfect." Sounds like a heavy burden to me. I'm not going to put that one on you.

For your part, you should stop trying to figure out the latest perfect eating advice to follow. It's just as futile as the people in the Old Testament trying to live perfectly by the Law. The prophet Jeremiah talked about God writing the Law on our hearts (Jer. 31:33). That's more like it.

Perhaps you have seen people who become so invested in eating only organic food and drinking only the cleanest water that they have no time to be a light in this world. They are so rigid about food and so fearful of polluting their bodies that people stop inviting them over to eat. They become so preachy about food that people stop wanting to talk to them. The all-consuming goal of their life becomes keeping their body as pure as possible. What's the point?

Jesus put things in perspective: "Don't you see that whatever enters the mouth goes into the stomach and then out of the body?" (Matt. 15:17, NIV). He is addressing the Jews about their obsessive attention to the rituals of avoiding unclean food, while at the same time they were speaking evil words.

On the flip side, the ancients had a saying: "Let us just eat and drink, for tomorrow we will die." (See Isaiah 22:13; Luke 12:19; 1 Corinthians 15:32.) I've heard people use that as an excuse even today. They say, "I could spend a bunch of time taking care of myself, and then I could be hit by a bus tomorrow. What's the point?"

A more pertinent question would be: What happens if you *don't* die tomorrow? Or even in ten years? What if you have to live with the effects of your abuse until you die at eighty-five? I've seen too many people who suffer from abuse-created ailments and who wish that they had taken better care of themselves early on. Was it worth it? Ask a diabetic with regard to sugar abuse or an emphysema sufferer with regard to smoking.

Bad Health Is Like Bad Debt

We need to figure out our priorities and stick with them. In general, the thrust of the medical system seems to be making sure that we all live a very long life. Quality of life is secondary to the length of the life. I strongly disagree with that. I believe that "running the race" with excellence should be our goal. In other words, while I'm here, I'm going to do what God is calling me to do. Therefore I need to have energy. I need to have good health. I do not want to blame my bad health for my inability to do things.

Truthfully, bad health is like debt. Both bad health and debt are bad masters. Debt makes you say, "I'm not sure I can offer help here. After all, I have a huge debt that I need to keep working on getting rid of." Bad health is similar.

We need health and wellness so that whenever God calls us to do something, we can answer the bell. Good health is a great testimony to God's goodness and provision.

I'm a big believer in the idea that we are responsible for doing and God is responsible for the results. If we do what God tells us, the results will be His responsibility. You can test it out. Lean on the Helper to show you what parts of the advice in this book are meant for you. Then, with His help, do those things. If you are not sure that you will "hear" God correctly, then let Him show you by the results.

God loves us. We do not need to coerce Him into helping us. We only need to pray for direction, do our part, and then let God do His part in His time.

Intuitively Healthy

I want you to learn how to live in your own body:

Not to take your health for granted

To listen to your body when it's dysfunctional

To be able to figure out your body's weaknesses and to be diligent in supporting those areas

To focus on the true problems instead of wasting time concentrating on areas of your body that rarely or never have problems

I want to make you intuitive about the health of your body. For instance, if someone says you need to do a colon cleanse, ask yourself, "Do I have problems with bowel movements or with signs and symptoms of toxicities? Do I have elevated liver enzymes? Constipation?" If not, don't waste your time, money, or effort on a problem that doesn't exist. Is your colon important? Sure. But so is your immune system. So is your heart. So is your brain.

Just focus on what the Holy Spirit says to focus on. Then you can rest in confidence. You don't need to worry about what you don't need to worry about.

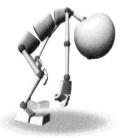

Chapter 4

HEALTHY EATING

Much of the food we eat today does not resemble the food that God created for us. In an attempt to make food more marketable and more palatable, we have made changes that have affected its nutritional value significantly. We wanted fluffier cakes, so we have them—and we are paying the price with our health. We have used our taste buds to tell us what foods to eat when we should have been asking our brains.

Our goal is to live a healthier lifestyle. Why is it as difficult for us to figure out how to eat healthier meals as it is to find the time to exercise? Somehow those two goals seem elusive.

Let's take a look at our most common excuses for not trying to improve our diets.

1. **"It costs too much money."** I'm not going to lie to you. It can cost more, but you can find ways to cut the expense. If you buy all organic food at the store, it's definitely going to cost you more. Health food can't compare to ramen noodles at five for a buck, a family-size box of mac and cheese for twenty cents more, the five frozen pizzas for ten dollars, or the ten-pound can of pork and beans from Costco.

   However, if you are committed to doing this, you can take steps to keep it cheaper. You can grow your own veggies, find local farmers who will sell you chickens that have been raised naturally, or go online and buy fifty-pound bags of spelt flour. Money should not be a barrier to good health.

When you eat healthier food, you will eat less of it. A slice of truly whole-grain bread will be more filling than two or three slices of Wonder Bread, and you will be less likely to overeat.

2. **"I don't have the time."** I do not buy this excuse. People complain how much more time it takes to cook regular oats compared to instant oats. Really? If I microwave a bowl of regular oats, it may take three minutes. The instant oatmeal cook time is one to two minutes. What kind of NASCAR world do you live in that you're worried about shaving sixty seconds off your morning preparations? Plus, then you can add whatever flavorings you want instead of the sugar and artificial stuff "they" decide belongs in your breakfast oatmeal.

I can throw a bag of frozen veggies and some ground turkey into a skillet and have it cooked up in less than five minutes. Really. I can make an omelet (and eat it) in less than five minutes. (OK, maybe I'm a bit embarrassed to admit that I can and do wolf down food that quickly. That's one of my food habits that I *don't* recommend following.)

I'm not asking you to pull out your Franklin Planner and set up two to three hours a day for meal preparation, although if you can, that's fine. My mother is awesome. She's a classic version of the 1960s' housewife. She plans. She's already looking into her next meal as soon as the dishes are finished for the current meal. I love her food, and she's an amazing cook. But in my home, we've never been able to be that meal-conscious. We are far more spontaneous.

You can do it either way. But I really don't want to hear how much time it takes.

3. **"I am afraid I won't like healthy foods."** This is the worst excuse of them all. Of course, ignoring a sense of one's own mortality and desire to be healthy, most people would pick a gooey chocolate chip cookie or a big frosting-covered cinnamon roll over brussels sprouts any day of the week. I know. I know. (Some of you "freaks" out there would actually prefer the brussels sprouts, and I'm proud of you. But you are definitely the exception and not the rule.)

For most of us, we need to link junky eating to an unwelcome outcome, such as being fat or sick or in pain or having nonstop diarrhea. Once we make the connection, we will modify our eating and drinking.

And once we make the switch, we will never look back. My patients actually say, "I drank a soda and, wow...it was way too sweet!" After a while your taste buds will start appreciating the nuances of real food and even come to prefer it.

4. **"It is easier to stop and pick up fast food on the way home from work."** I try to tell my patients that they just need to plan ahead, and if they fail to plan, they can still go through the drive-through on the way home. You just make different choices.

Instead of getting the Big Mac and fries, you can order the grilled chicken and eat it without the bun; you can also get a salad and maybe even a mini-bag of carrots or an apple. Or you can go to the local Mexican fast-food place and order a crunchy taco fresco style (no cheese).

My guess is that you really want to go the fast-food place not so much because it's fast, but because you want to indulge your desire for junk food. But if you've truly forgotten and you're really "stuck," you do have those options.

The USDA Pyramid Scheme

In April of 2005, the United States Department of Agriculture (USDA) released a new food guidance scheme based on the 2005 *Dietary Guidelines for Americans*. This replaced the previous pyramid scheme from the 1990s. The old pyramid recommended eating six to eleven servings of grains a day. This, of course, is fabulous for farmers who are trying to make a living selling grain. However, for the rest of us, it means obesity. Here are some of the highlights from the new pyramid scheme:

Grains

We are supposed to aim for eating at least half of the grains as "whole grains." So, according to the USDA, what is the other half supposed to be? Bleached white flour (processed from wheat) that has been enriched with the nutrients that were stripped from it in the bleaching process. Another common substitute for whole grains is quick-cooking white rice, which is almost entirely starch with the outer covering of bran totally removed. "Whole-wheat flour" is not whole wheat. The wheat germ has been taken out because the germ layer contains oils that would go rancid on the shelves after the flour is ground. If you truly want whole-wheat flour, you need to grind your own or watch as someone grinds it for you.

In Bible times, bread was considered the staff of life for two good reasons: the grains were not genetically altered or stripped of their fiber and nutrient-dense germ layer, and also because the people walked wherever they went. Back then, everyone's job was physical. They ate because they needed to, and they burned it off before the next meal.

Unlike our ancestors, we Americans do very little exercise. So what foods should we continue to eat if we want to make sure that we become nice and fat for the slaughter? Cakes, cookies, crackers, popcorn, English muffins, bagels, muffins, pasta, pancakes, waffles, most buns and breads, and so forth.

Milk

The USDA would have us believe that dairy products are the only calcium-rich foods available and therefore are critical to your health. Of course they are referring to pasteurized milk products. The truth is that milk is not a great source of calcium for a number of people. I know that contradicts the "Milk: it does a body good" promo campaign.

In Appendix C, "Dr. B's Suggestions" (at the end of the book), I have provided a list of calcium-containing foods. I think you'll be amazed at how many foods besides milk can easily provide your calcium needs. If you still feel you need additional calcium, I have also provided a list of good-quality calcium supplements there.

I am a big fan of raw milk, and I am writing this from the dairy state of Wisconsin, where it is illegal to sell raw milk and raw milk products (like cheese) in the stores. For the first half of the twentieth century, raw milk was still easy to obtain throughout the country. Then pasteurization of milk became mandatory because of the bacterial infections unpasteurized milk could cause. However, pasteurization requires heat, which destroys not only bacteria but also enzymes such as lactase and heat-sensitive proteins. These enzymes assist the human body in processing the large proteins present in milk: casein and lactalbumin (whey).

I would estimate that 85 percent of the patients who come to my office for food allergy testing turn out to be sensitive to pasteurized dairy products, while only 20 percent are sensitive to raw dairy products.

Why am I going into all of this? Isn't this book supposed to be about improving how your thyroid functions? Correct. And proper thyroid function depends upon keeping your body's inflammation at a reasonable level. Food allergies and sensitivities create inflammation, and that can definitely hinder your thyroid from functioning properly.

Besides milk sensitivities, 95 percent of the patients I have tested have sensitivities to bleached flour, and about 90 percent have sensitivities to sugar and high-fructose corn syrup. (This may not be a good representation of the rest of society since I see many patients who are already sick and who have been to other medical professionals before they come to me.) Still, the road signs are obvious: eat natural, unprocessed food to keep your body healthy.

No-No Foods

I strongly urge you to eliminate from your diet all types of white flour, pasteurized dairy products, artificial sweetening products, all chemically processed oils, and all genetically modified foods.

White flour

Eliminate enriched bleached (and even unbleached) white wheat flour from your diet. Flour products include cakes, muffins, cookies, crackers, pancakes, waffles, pasta, bread, breaded and deep-fried products, English muffins, and bagels, as well as gravies and sauces (with flour as a thickener).

I know. I know. That's everything you eat. I've heard that before. Here's the other thing I hear often: "Don't worry; I eat whole-wheat pasta and whole-wheat bread." Unfortunately, those have processed flour in them too. Don't believe me? Go to the grocery store and take a look at the ingredient labels on all the breads. They all have one or more of the following: enriched flour, unbleached flour, flour, wheat flour, white flour, etc. It's probably easier to just eliminate all wheat products than to explain to you what you specifically need to eliminate.

The only bread that I am confident in recommending to you is Ezekiel 4:9 Bread. Two reasons: first, the recipe derives from God's prophetic word to Ezekiel. (He was told to protest against Israel by lying first on one side for half a year and then on the other side for half a year, cooking this bread over cow dung. But don't worry; the Food for Life people who make Ezekiel 4:9 Bread have a different baking method.)

Second, not only do they avoid processed flour, but also they sprout the grain first. This means that the first part of the process is to lay out a bunch of seed/grain and then add water. Within a short period of time, the grain begins to sprout. As soon as it does so, the water gets drained off, the sprouted grain gets dried out, and then it gets ground into flour. Once it starts to sprout, it is now part grain and part vegetable plant stem. People who have allergies to grains (which, unfortunately, is a fairly large slice of the American pie) do not react to bread made with sprouted grains as much (or at all) compared to how they would react to typical white or "whole-grain" bread.

In contrast, how does the flour industry process the wheat kernel? The three-step process begins with the removal of the germ, which contains vital oils, vitamins, and minerals. Most "whole-wheat flours" are actually degermed ground wheat. The wheat germ is removed because it's the most sensitive to spoilage and rancidity. Consequently, once it has been removed, the flour can last almost indefinitely on the shelf.

After the germ has been removed, the final step takes the remaining endosperm and bleaches it. Yes, that's right. With chemical bleaching agents. This process makes the flour whiter and fluffier.

Generations used to process white flour this way for years until they recognized that people were getting sick. People had become deficient in the B vitamins formerly provided by the germ of the wheat kernel. Instead of saying, "Oops. We made a mistake. That was dumb. Let's stop processing the flour," people wanted to have their cake and eat it too (pun intended). So they returned the vitamins they had taken out of the flour, in the form of synthetic vitamins made from coal tar, and now they called the flour "enriched"—as if somehow they had done the flour a favor. I'm sure the makers of angel food cakes and sandwich breads praised this as a "breakthrough," but it has brought down a curse of problems on what used to be called the staff of life.

So let's get this straight. Bread in grocery stores, restaurants, and bakeries contains processed flour—even most of the "whole-wheat" breads, and they can cause problems just as white flour can. Also, pastas not specifically made from another grain (such as rice pasta, spelt pasta, or quinoa pasta) can cause problems. Semolina, durum, and graham are wheat derivatives, thus included in the no-no category. I know a lot of people say that spelt and kamut are types of wheat; however, they are ancient grains that have not been extensively genetically modified. My patients tend to test better on them than most other wheat grains.

Genetically modified foods

The Bible tells us to not cross-pollinate grains. (See Leviticus 19:19, which speaks about not cross-fertilizing two kinds of plants or cross-breeding different kinds of animals.) This avoids a problem that agricultural scientists call "genetic drift."

However, when scientists, in their effort to discover new ways to grow enough food for the world, discovered how to mix and match the features of plants and animals, they may have improved the economics of farming, but they opened a Pandora's box of new problems. Many of our food sensitivities and allergies relate to our most genetically altered crops, such as wheat, corn, soy, oranges, and more.

We have genetically modified corn so that it can be sprayed with a strong herbicide from Monsanto called Roundup and the corn plant is not harmed at all, while all the weeds are killed.[1] I don't know about you, but I find this kind of information scary. I do not believe that Roundup-resistant corn was on God's seven-day to-do list. (Nor was it an inadvertent omission.)

The genetically modified corn we feed to our cattle is meant to produce nice fat animals in the shortest period of time in order to maximize the rancher's profits. It used to take two to three years for a cow to be ready for slaughter. The current feed gets the cow ready in approximately six months. Some experts have suggested that if these cows were not taken to market as soon as they are, they would die of obesity-related disease within nine to twelve months.

I believe we were made to eat only the meat, seeds, veggies, fruits, beans, and grains that God put on the earth and told us would be safe to eat, and that we have been reaping the consequences of our interference with His master plan.

Pasteurized dairy products

This includes pasteurized milk and cream as well as cheese, yogurt, sour cream, cottage cheese, kefir, and anything made from pasteurized milk. Pasteurization was intended to solve gastrointestinal ailments that arose from the consumption of raw milk. I'm sure that poor handling of the milk and the resulting contamination of the milk with fecal bacteria was largely to blame. And yet not everyone suffered from raw milk consumption. If everyone had experienced problems with the raw milk, then it would have made sense to insist on across-the-board pasteurization.

The other aspect of pasteurization is shelf life. As with other natural foods, raw milk has a shorter shelf life than pasteurized milk. You can't expect it to last in your fridge for three weeks (as perhaps you've done with pasteurized milk) without spoilage.

We do have some Christians who object that we are the only species that drinks the milk of another species, as if this explains why so many of us have problems with dairy products. They say this proves that we were never meant to consume dairy products. I disagree with them. In the Bible, no lesser men than David and Jesus consumed "curds," which is cheese. (See 2 Samuel 17:29; Isaiah 7:15.) And why would God promise His people a land flowing with milk and honey if milk was bad for them? (The milk in those days would not have been pasteurized, by the way.)

Despite my warnings about dairy products, I tell my patients that butter is OK. How can this be true, since butter is made from milk? This is because the composition of butter is primarily milk fat with a small amount of milk protein in it. (A product called ghee or clarified butter takes out the remaining milk protein.) Since milk proteins and lactose are the usual sources of problems for most individuals, butter typically does not make a person with dairy sensitivities react. Of course, butter is a fat that is dense with calories, so people who are trying to lose weight should keep that in mind.

Processed and synthetic sweeteners

I love sweets probably more than most of you. When I was younger, I used to pour sugar (you might think I meant to write "sprinkle," but I mean *pour* because we had an old Tupperware sugar container that had a spout on one side) on my hot or cold cereal in the morning. I used so much so that I would have spoonfuls of that gritty goodness in the bottom of my bowl; I used to spoon up milk and granulated sugar once I was out of cereal. I was a sugar nut.

Now, it's true that God made your taste buds so that sweetness would guide you to good foods. The Book of Proverbs provides this advice about honey:

> My son, eat honey, for it is good,
> Yes, the honey from the comb is sweet to your taste.
> —PROVERBS 24:13

If you find honey, eat just enough—
too much of it, and you will vomit.

—Proverbs 25:16, niv

It is not good to eat too much honey.

—Proverbs 25:27, niv

As you can see, honey is good, but too much is not good. Molasses, maple syrup (the real stuff from a tree, not the corn syrup that has been artificially flavored with maple that you find labeled as "syrup" on most grocery store shelves), and other sweeteners in nature are typically fine too if consumed in moderation. In each of these cases, the syrups contain sugars but also enzymes, minerals, and nutrients that the body needs to process the sugar.

The problem with white table sugar and high-fructose corn syrup is that they are so purified. Sugar is more than 99 percent sucrose. All the nutrients in the cane plant have been removed. (The "nutritional waste product" is called molasses.) I do understand the reason for doing this. Refined sugar can serve as a far more effective sweetener in a wider variety of applications. It carries no flavor or aftertaste. As pure sweetness, it complements everything. It can sweeten cinnamon, mints, or chocolate without changing the essence of each.

But what else does it do? Refined sugar makes so many foods so cheap and appealing that Western civilization has become addicted to it. Have you ever heard of a molasses addict or a honey addict? Neither have I. But we live in a society of more sugar addicts, soda addicts, and obese (often also diabetic) individuals than anywhere else in the world.

Then there are the artificial sweeteners. Food should not be made in a chemistry lab. I believe that artificial sweeteners should be avoided—all of them. This includes the following:

+ Splenda (sucralose)

+ NutraSweet (aspartame)

+ Acesulfame-K

+ Saccharin

+ Other artificial sweeteners such as neotame and cyclamate

+ And any new ones that come along

If the chemical composition of these sweeteners act like the pesticides with which they shares similarities (see Appendix B), then many of the problems will not fully peak for decades because cancer may be the cumulative, devastating outcome. The widespread use of artificial sweeteners provides a societal real-time study. All of you who are using artificial sweeteners have signed up to participate in this study to measure the toxicity of these chemicals on the human population. You are a guinea pig, a lab rat. You can, however, resign from the study by banning artificial sweeteners from your diet.

Artificial sweeteners may appear where you least expect them. In the past several years, as people have tried to avoid artificial sweeteners while still trying to lower their carbohydrates and caloric intake, they have looked more at that part of the food label. Read the whole list. You might be surprised sometimes. If you see ingredients on a food label that you have a hard time recognizing, do not buy that food item.

For example, one day I was looking for hot cocoa mix. I had the choice of two brands. One brand had a sugar-free version, which I knew I didn't want, and it also had two "regular" flavors: milk chocolate and dark chocolate. I bought the milk chocolate flavor and tried it at home. It tasted as if it had artificial sweeteners in it. I thought, "Man, I bought the wrong kind." (I'm known for looking so carefully at something and then picking up the can next to it, assuming it is the same.) So I thought it was my fault. I looked more carefully at the can. *Hmm…* It was not the sugar-free version. I turned to the ingredient label. First ingredient: sugar…then dry milk, then cocoa…so far so good. I read all the way down the list until, way at the bottom, I read "sucralose," which, of course, is Splenda. I was confused. Why on earth would they put *both* sugar and artificial sweetener in the same product? I called the company to find out. Their representative indicated that since sucralose is so intensely sweet, they could add less volume of sweetener to each scoop and therefore they could give the customer more cups of hot cocoa with each can. They couldn't see my point that there are a lot of people who do not want artificial sweeteners and think they are unhealthy.

They have not changed the formula as far as I know. So I've gone with the other brand since then. Certainly it makes more sense to make up your own hot chocolate mix using rice milk or almond milk, cocoa powder, and some xylitol or stevia as a natural, low-carbohydrate sweetener.

Salt

I realize this is the no-no list, but generally, I'm OK with salt. I usually recommend sea salt because that's how people initially found and used it. I have a problem with my patients eating salt only if they know they have a problem with salt. I know salt isn't evil because the Bible talks about us being as valuable as salt. "You are the salt of the earth" (Matt. 5:13).

Many of my patients suffer with low blood pressure, so I recommend sea salt when they crave salt. I believe that their bodies are telling them to increase their salt intake to elevate their blood pressure. I also believe that some people are sensitive to sodium, which often happens because of a calcium deficiency. I recommend that those people increase their intake of calcium, magnesium, and sometimes potassium.

Margarine or shortening

These are oils that have been chemically altered. I have suggested for years that Promise, Country Crock, Crisco, and the like are not foods. They are chemical substances made to be like food. Recent studies on trans fats have begun to prove my concerns. Years from now we will realize that when these fats enter the human system and become absorbed in the same way that butter, oils, and animal fats are, the human body does not know what to do with them because it was never meant to eat them. We will find that they are one of the culprits behind obesity, neurological diseases, and even heart attacks.

The terrible thing about this is that since these were oils at one time, people have assumed that they could not have the same negative impact believed to come from saturated fats. But these oils have been saturated by bubbling hydrogen through them, and they have become more like lard and butter than they are like oils.

What are you supposed to use in place of these fake oils? My first recommendation is olive oil. If you need something that is a solid at room temperature, not an oil, choose butter. I would even prefer lard over these fake fats. Some other good oils are gaining popularity, such as grape seed oil and walnut oil, which can be fine when not overly purified or processed.

I link all the remaining oils together (canola, safflower, corn, and sunflower). Many people think that canola oil is good because it is monosaturated (like olive oil), but canola oil, made from rapeseed, has had to undergo a great deal of processing to make it store-ready. The more processing something requires, the more I try to avoid it. Processing oils leaves a lot of free radicals (especially with the polyunsaturated oils), which can damage the circulatory system and heart and possibly induce cancer cells to multiply. Some people use virgin coconut oil. I don't have any red flags with that one, so if it seems to help you and you enjoy cooking with it, go ahead.

If you learn nothing else from reading this book, learn this: food should not be made in a (where?)...right...chemistry lab!

Do You Have a Wheat Allergy?

Many people are checked for gluten sensitivity with a lab test. They come in saying they had the gluten test (Anti-Gliadin Antibody Assay) and it was negative. Then I check them. "Well," I say, "you're sensitive to wheat."

They don't understand it. "So I am sensitive to gluten?"

"No."

They stare at me confused. "Huh? How is that possible?"

Because wheat is more than gluten, that's how.

There's the bran (outer covering). There's the germ (the stored nutrients). Finally, there's the endosperm. The endosperm has proteins and starches in it. This is the main part of most flours, and it does contain gluten. (Gluten is the elastic protein that is left behind after we remove the starch part of the wheat. It makes for fluffy angel food cakes, and it allows us to squeeze our white bread until it compresses back into a dough ball.)

Gluten is comprised of two main groups of proteins: gliadins and glutenins. Because these are proteins, the gastrointestinal system breaks them down first into polypeptides or peptide chains (smaller chunks of protein-like beads of pearls, but still composed of several amino acids). If digestion is incomplete, it's possible to absorb these pieces of protein. When the blood system "sees" one of these peptides, it can mistakenly view it as an intruder and form an immunological reaction (allergy) to it.

From that point on, the body will begin making antibodies specifically geared to attack and destroy that peptide every time it enters the system. Complete digestion in a healthy gastrointestinal tract would break these proteins down all the way into their smallest units, amino acids. The body doesn't form reactions to amino acids, because it knows what they are. They are vital building blocks to enable the body to make proteins that become cartilage, skin, bone, organs, and blood vessels.

It is thought that one type of peptide that contains nineteen amino acids strung together in a specific sequence is a culprit in celiac disease, which is gastrointestinal erosion from repeated reactions with this protein fragment of gluten. So labs designed a test to identify this antibody to this one polypeptide.

I know that the above information sounds pretty complicated, but I'm trying to say this: Isn't it possible that since there are probably millions of ways that this long string of beads (hundreds long) called gluten could be broken down, that therefore other smaller pieces could also cause the body's immune system to hyper-react with inflammation? The answer, of course, is *yes*.

This is why, of course, it's OK to have the blood test to determine if you have allergies to wheat and other gluten-containing products—but also why a negative test does not preclude the diagnosis of wheat allergies/sensitivities.

A good, commonsense way for you to find out is to "eat clean," avoiding items that commonly produce food allergies or sensitivities such as grains, dairy, sweets, and so forth. And then once you feel good (which I think you will after eating clean for a month), you can bring single foods back one at a time to see if you react. I tell people to plan on a whole day of eating a lot of what they eliminated.

Two questions will be answered: Do you react? If so, what was the reaction? The reaction could be right at the time of eating, minutes or hours after eating, or even the next day. If you experience diarrhea within thirty minutes of your first meal with that food, please don't torture yourself by continuing to eat that food the rest of the day. You just got your answer. Once you have your answers, write them all down in a notebook, and then eat "clean" again for a few more days until you have no remnant of the previous reaction; then introduce the next food. I usually tell patients to make sure they pick days to do these food challenges when they do not necessarily need to feel good or be productive. I don't want them to expect to go to work and have to run to the bathroom every fifteen minutes.

This is called the elimination-provocation diet. It allows you to diagnosis your own allergies and sensitivities. The only two downsides of this approach are: One, it is very time-consuming; it can take a good year to evaluate fifty plus foods. Secondly, it doesn't effectively evaluate substances that are not foods or that do not cause sudden reactions. For instance, inhaling benzene or using certain additives in toothpaste or cleaners may cause cancer over several years or decades of using them. Will they show a reaction during a single day of exposure? Probably not. Many of these items progressively annoy the body but won't show up in the short term.

However, at this phase I'm more concerned with having you clean up these items that are causing symptoms now and less concerned with the long-term effect of certain other foods or products.

Different grains are just that—different. Treat them all individually. Barley is not wheat, and wheat is not oats, and so forth. Even though they are wheat species, I still treat grains like bulgur, Kamut, and spelt as different grains. But I treat graham, semolina, and durum flour as refined wheat derivatives. Buckwheat, by the way, is not wheat. Most people do not react to buckwheat or rye flours, although both of them are pretty strongly flavored to cook with unless you're using them as a secondary ingredient or you just really love the flavor of buckwheat or rye.

I like whole-grain spelt as a substitute for white wheat flour in recipes. If a recipe calls for two cups of enriched flour, you can add two cups of whole-grain spelt in its place. It will not be as fluffy and soft as enriched flour, but it also won't be brick-hard. It carries a very slight but pleasant flavor. Still, if spelt causes similar symptoms as wheat products, then just stop using it. Also—please, please, please do *not* buy white spelt flour. Why? Because once we go down that road and everyone realizes that spelt is less allergenic than wheat, people will soon start bleaching and genetically altering spelt—and we'll be right back where we started. Choose only whole-grain spelt for that reason.

What You *Should* Eat

Up to now I have been trying to keep you from eating food that is potentially inflammatory to your system. Since, however, you have most likely picked up this book because you want help with your low-functioning thyroid gland, here are some recommendations regarding your diet.

In general, as you may have heard it said, "shop the outside (perimeter)" of the store layout—produce, seafood, meats. The supposed timesaving of the pre-packaged foods aren't worth the health hassles. Beyond that, here is my advice:

Fresh and frozen vegetables

No canned veggies, please. They've been cooked too much. That leaves fresh and frozen vegetables, and there is a debate as to which is better for you. You may wonder why. Most of us would assume that fresh vegetables are better than anything that has been frozen.

But here's the thinking: frozen vegetables are picked, flash-frozen, and packed within a short period of time and then shipped frozen to the grocery store. They have had the chance to ripen on the vine, and they are almost as fresh as the day they were picked. In-store fresh vegetables are often equally fresh when the produce is in season, but some fruits and vegetables have been shipped from around world. In order to ship them so that they will be ready to sell, many need to be picked before they are ripe. They ripen in transit, or, in some cases, they receive a dose of ethylene gas in the warehouse to ripen them. This is why many store tomatoes are more pink than red. (Speaking of tomatoes, you should know that tomato products are fine when they're canned. They lose some of their nutrients, but they remain high in carotenoids and lutein even when they have been diced, crushed, stewed, made into sauce.)

Many vegetables lose their labile (unstable) vitamins such as B vitamins and ascorbic acid in the freezing process, but those would have been lost in the cooking process anyway.

Deli meat

Deli meats are certainly not perfect food, but they are better than gorging on bread, muffins, and pasta salad. When people feel stuck with regard to controlling their eating, I give them permission to grab some deli meat, especially if they are having a hard time getting enough protein in their diet.

I know what you're thinking: "How am I supposed to eat my deli meat without bread?" Answer: roll it up and eat it like a carrot. Or, if you're having bakery cravings, you can imagine that it's a bread stick.

Nuts and seeds

Unless you have an allergy to nuts (and you may not be allergic to all nuts), consider nuts as a source of protein. Almonds, walnuts, pecans, cashews, peanuts (really a legume), hazelnuts, chestnuts, macadamia nuts, and less-common types of nuts can supply protein and other nutrients in an unprocessed form. Don't forget about the many types of edible seeds, some of which you can eat by the handful, such as sunflower seeds, pumpkin seeds, and pine nuts.

Beans and legumes

Technically soft seeds, beans and legumes have been staples of good nutrition for centuries. Most of them come dried, so you will need to reconstitute them and cook them, but you can also buy many of them canned simply in water with a little salt. Lentils (the "fast food" of legumes, because they cook quickly), chickpeas, pinto beans, kidney beans, lima beans, great northern beans, etc. can be used in such a wide variety of recipes that you will never be bored with them.

Nut butters

Again, for those of you who are having massive hunger pains and you can't figure out what to eat, how about peanut butter or almond butter or even cashew butter? Here come the questions again (I can hear them after twenty years in practice): "How am I supposed to eat peanut butter if you won't allow me jelly and I can't put it on bread?" First of all, quit sassing me. Second, you have a lot of options. You could just stick a spoon into the peanut butter jar and spoon it right into your mouth. Or you could be like me and add a bit of honey on the top of the peanut butter. Or you could still add jelly to your spoonful of peanut butter—as long as it is the fruit-juice-sweetened kind (one example is Simply Fruit). Or you could use a celery stick or yummy apple slices to scoop up the peanut butter.

Warning: Commercial peanut butter has had its oil hydrogenated like margarine, and then, to make it even more yummy, sugar has been added. The peanut butter you should look for can be found on the same shelf as the other stuff, but it should say "natural peanut butter" on the label. If you still aren't sure, look for the peanut oil floating on top of it. No (sigh), I'm not suggesting that you eat peanut-oil-drippy peanut butter. Just open it up when you get home and mix it around with a spoon or a knife until the oil gets stirred in. With the oil stirred in, store the peanut butter in the fridge to keep it from separating again. Some stores carry natural peanut butter in the refrigerated section (typically near the butter, chocolate chip cookie dough, and yogurt) that does not need to be stirred because of the refrigeration.

And yes, you might like one of the other types of nut butters. Almond butter is tasty, and almonds are a good source of protein and healthy fats. Cashew butter is a personal favorite of mine. Tahini is sesame seed butter. I'm not a big fan, but some people really like it. It's also good for you. Hummus recipes use tahini along with garbanzo beans (also called chickpeas). Hummus and tahini are very healthy "butters," rich in protein and nutrients.

What Should You Drink?

I firmly believe that when you are thirsty, you should drink water. Your body thrives on it. None of us need soft drinks, alcohol, tea, coffee, or even juice to quench thirst. We need pure water.

Of course that brings us to the issue of how to find pure water, doesn't it? Health professionals and nutritionists will give you a number of differing responses. Let's go through some of the options:

Municipal tap water

This is water that has been treated to remove all living organisms (bacteria, parasites, etc.) and particulate matter. Using aluminum sulfate, the water purification process causes impurities to coagulate so that they can be more easily filtered and removed as the particulate settles. This process is called coagulation or flocculation. To assist in the sterilization of the water, chlorine is added.

However, the disinfection with chlorine can cause problems. According to the Centers for Disease Control and Prevention: "Disinfection by-products (DBPs), also called trihalomethanes, are formed when chlorine and bromine interact with natural organic materials in water, such as in chlorinated drinking water and chlorine-treated swimming pools.... People are exposed to DBPs by drinking chlorinated or brominated water and by breathing in air containing DBPs. The skin also absorbs DBPs during bathing and swimming."[2]

The potential carcinogenicity of these compounds necessitates regular monitoring of the municipal water systems. "The human health effects from DBPs at low environmental exposures are unknown. Humans exposed to unusually large amounts of some DBPs could experience liver damage and decreased nervous system activity."[3]

Chlorine is a powerful oxidant and fairly inexpensive, which makes it great for use in municipal water systems. However, I believe that hydrogen peroxide and ozone will eventually take over as the primarily sterilization agent in water treatment plants in the United States. Both are very strong oxidants (which means they will destroy or kill anything with which they come in contact). What's better, hydrogen peroxide is simply H_2O_2, which means it breaks down into oxygen (O_2) and water (H_2O). In the case of ozone, it is simply O_3 (three atoms of oxygen stuck together). Once ozone does its job, it breaks down into stable oxygen gas, which has only two oxygen atoms stuck together.

What else is added to municipal water supplies? Fluoride. This is probably the most controversial of all the aspects of our municipal water supply. If you're a dentist, you probably are quite adamant that this is a good thing. After all, it helps make the enamel of the teeth stronger and decreases cavities. On the other hand, fluoride is not a nutrient. In fact, for the most part, fluoride is a toxin—a poison. Too much can cause a condition known as fluorosis. Dental fluorosis happens due to exposure to fluoride while teeth are developing. It can cause anything from white spots or streaks to dark mottling of the teeth. Skeletal fluorosis from excessive exposure to fluoride results in pain or damage to bones and joints. In addition to the fluorosis concern, over one hundred studies show lower IQ levels with humans and animals that have been exposed to fluoride. For this reason, many countries are no longer fluoridating their water.

Many of the most popular home water purification systems, such as Brita and Pur, do not remove fluoride or chloride from the water. There are two water purification systems that I prefer.

Distilled water

It's the cheapest of the options. You are basically using a distilling unit to boil your water into steam and then allowing it to condense back into water and having that "distilled" water drip into a collection container. The idea is that any minerals and materials with a different boiling point than water will not end up in the collection container.

Critics will complain that distilled water is very acidic water, but the truth is, it's neutral. It hasn't melted from the mountaintops and then poured down a mountain stream picking up minerals from the rocks along the way. It also has not come from between two layers of bedrock, again assimilating minerals from the adjacent rocks.

The benefit of minerals in our water is that they have an alkalinizing effect on our bodies to counter all the acidifying processed food that we eat. This is why you hear people touting mineral water or spring water. But there are two problems with that. One is that most of the spring (or artesian) water sold in bottles is just water from the tap. It might originate in a deep spring or a good water source, but it's been fluoridated and chlorinated, which are two of the reasons you are trying to purify your water in the first place. The other flaw of the bottled spring water is that, along with all the good minerals, there's no guarantee that you're also not getting a bunch of other minerals and pollutants in the water. We've been such bad stewards of our environment over the years that we still have DDT showing up in our food supply.

Some of you might say, "Well, that was a long time ago. We're much better now in protecting our water supply today." Really? This is from an Associated Press article entitled "Drugs Found in Drinking Water" in *USA Today*. The article begins, "A vast array of pharmaceuticals—including antibiotics, anti-convulsants, mood stabilizers and sex hormones—have been found in the drinking water supplies of at least 41 million Americans, an Associated Press investigation shows."[4]

How is this getting in our water supply? One way is from water runoff from farms and ranches. Over half of all antibiotics made in this country end up being given to livestock to keep them from getting sick. (Believe me, that's a problem for more than just our water supply.) Much of the rest comes from the medications that people's bodies do not fully absorb, which are shed in their urine and stools and which cannot be completely eliminated in water-purification processes. Still others come from the extra medications that people dispose of by flushing them down the toilet.

Reverse osmosis (RO)

In this system of water purification, minerals are selectively removed from the water. The process removes both good minerals such as calcium, magnesium, and zinc as well as bad minerals such as lead, mercury, and aluminum. Aquafina and Dasani purify their water this way. You will find machines in stores to which you can bring your own jugs and fill them with machine-dispensed RO water for about twenty-five to forty cents. This may be pure enough.

However, one of my patients who had been having bothersome stomach pains brought in several types of water, and we tested her on all of them. She reacted to the distilled water, the store RO water, and to tap water. She did not react to the deep spring water in our community (Petrifying Springs). It turns out that she was reacting to the chlorine in the water supply.

If she were to use a straight RO system, she would have trouble. RO systems remove only minerals, not other pollutants. So along with an RO filter system, she had to use a three- or four-stage filtration system. This combines the benefits of reverse osmosis with a 5-micron sediment filter to eliminate particles with a charcoal filter. Charcoal filters are good at taking tastes and smells out of the water (absorption happens as with baking soda), and they are also good at removing the fluoride and chloride compounds from the water.

You can find countertop or under-the-sink models for less than five hundred dollars. I use a portable three-step filter that I connect to my laundry tub in the basement, where I fill five-gallon jugs to use at home and at the clinic. The type that I have is made by Pure Earth Technologies and costs less than two hundred dollars.[5] It does require filter replacement annually or biannually, so it is more expensive to maintain than a distiller.

Multistage reverse osmosis units and water distillers are meant to mimic rainwater. There are no minerals in rainwater. It is pure water, because it evaporates up into the sky and comes down as rain or snow.

If you are concerned about not getting enough vital minerals because of removing them out of your water supply, you should know, first of all, that most water does not provide very much in the way of minerals. You could probably take one good multimineral supplement pill per week, and you'd receive more minerals than you would all week in your water.

In the alternative realm, someone always claims to have the latest and greatest breakthrough, and this includes water purity. I do not recommend the screw-on faucet filter attachments, nor do I recommend the gravity filters such as Brita. I don't think they remove enough of the problematic pollutants in tap water. Ultraviolet light only sterilizes water. After ultraviolet treatment, chemicals remain in the water.

A few other new water treatment systems include some that, at this phase, I consider faddish, such as magnetic water treatment, ionizers, and energetic water systems.

You need pure water, essential for life, in order to function effectively. When you are thirsty, skip the soda, coffee, tea, vitamin water, Gatorade, Powerade, and even fruit juices. A refreshing glass of pure water is always best.

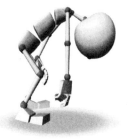

Chapter 5

IS YOUR THYROID AN UNDERACHIEVER?

Your butterfly-shaped thyroid gland is located in the front of your lower neck, just below your Adam's apple. As one of your largest endocrine glands, its primary function is to secrete hormones. By means of these hormones, your thyroid controls your metabolism, creates proteins, and sensitizes your body to other hormones.

The most important hormone made and secreted by your thyroid is known as thyroxine, better known as T4. On a biochemical level, a T4 molecule consists of the amino acid L-tyrosine with four iodine atoms attached to it, hence the T4 designation. In your body, an enzyme lops off one of the iodine atoms, leaving three still attached and creating a hormone known as triiodothyronine, also called T3. (Your thyroid manufactures some T3, but it releases an estimated twenty times more T4 than it does T3.) For factual purposes, we should note that the enzyme that removes the iodine atom also does it two more times, creating T2 and T1, but the levels and activity of these hormones are so insignificant that most of the medical community ignore them. However, T3 is significant. It is several times more bioactive than T4.

Collectively, these substances are known as thyroid hormone. They are essential for your nerve development, sexual development, and physical growth as well as for regulating your metabolic rate, your body heat, and your energy level.

Your thyroid gland depends on other glands in order to know when and when not to secrete more thyroid hormone. The hypothalamus gland is one of them. Almond-sized and located just below the thalamus above the brain stem, the hypothalamus gland communicates in two ways: (1) via the "electrical cords" we call nerves, which are made up of elongated cells called neurons, and (2) through blood proteins and steroids called hormones. For our purposes in this chapter, we're going to talk primarily about hormones.

Hormones, made and secreted by glands, make contact with hormonal receptors in cells, which stimulate those cells (and therefore the organ or gland made up of those cells) to function in a certain way. The more a particular hormone gets released, the more a particular function will occur in your body.

Your hypothalamus releases hormones that affect your body temperature, hunger, thirst, fatigue, and sleep. We're going to concentrate on how the hypothalamus affects your thyroid function, since that is the topic of this book. Your hypothalamus, when it detects the need for additional thyroid hormone, releases thyrotropin-releasing hormone (TRH). This hormone activates certain cells in the front part (anterior) of your pituitary gland to release thyroid-stimulating hormone (TSH). TSH then activates your thyroid, stimulating it to make and secrete additional thyroid hormone directly into your bloodstream.

Among other factors, your hypothalamus gland adjusts its activity according to the prevailing temperature of your environment. Have you ever wondered why, in the middle of a cold winter, you can go outdoors without a coat when the temperature is a "warm" 45°F, but you want to put on a parka if it's 45°F in the middle of summer? This happens because your hypothalamus has adjusted your body's thermostat to help it maintain a comfortable temperature. And your body's heating system is directly controlled by the activity of thyroid hormones circulating in your bloodstream. The more thyroid hormone you have in your circulatory system, the more heat your body will generate.

Along these lines, if your body is fighting an infection, agents in the bloodstream called pyrogens will stimulate the hypothalamus to cause a fever. The fever's purpose is to make your body an uncomfortable place for the foreign invaders, essentially to create an overheated environment in which it will be more difficult for them to multiply. This is why you shouldn't reach for a fever-reducing drug at the first sign of a fever. A recent clinical report from the American Academy of Pediatrics, in a reversal of years of pediatric practice, advises restraint in the use of antipyretics (medicines that can lower fevers) with regard to infections. One of the main antipyretics doctors recommend is acetaminophen. It's best to allow the fever to do its work unimpeded, both to fight the current infection and to build up resistance to future infections.[1]

One of the symptoms of hyperthyroidism (when excess thyroid hormone has been produced and secreted) is an elevated body temperature. Conversely, one of the symptoms of low thyroid function (hypothyroidism) is a low body temperature. We will discuss both hypothyroidism and hyperthyroidism in much more depth in the following pages.

Key Indicators of Hypothyroidism

Worldwide, hypothyroidism, or low thyroid function, is greatly underdiagnosed. One of the reasons for this is that so many of its symptoms are so commonplace. In fact, I dislike going through a list of hypothyroid symptoms with patients since they tend to rule out the diagnosis if they do not feel that they manifest all of them or even most of them, or if they have assumed that the symptoms came from another cause.

In truth, a hypothyroid patient might be able to identify only one or two signs or symptoms of an underfunctioning thyroid gland. The classic general hypothyroidism manifestations include fatigue, inability to lose weight (or gaining weight easily), intolerance to cold, and swelling (usually in the extremities: hands, lower legs, and feet).

Fatigue

The fatigue of hypothyroidism is not so much like the type of fatigue that results from heavy exertion, such as from rushing through a large airport carrying bulky suitcases, exercising long and hard at the gym, or walking up several flights of stairs. That type of fatigue resembles anemia (low oxygen to your body and brain). Neither is the fatigue like the chronic feeling of needing to take a nap in the middle of the afternoon, which I described in chapter 2 as typical of adrenal fatigue. Rather, the fatigue that comes from low thyroid function generally feels like exhaustion or tiredness all day long—morning, noon, and night. Some may describe it as sluggishness; for others it may come across as apathy.

Weight problems

Gaining weight and the inability to lose weight are challenging problems. Men and women both struggle with this, but more hypothyroid women seem to have weight struggles than hypothyroid men. I think it must be because men have much higher levels of testosterone in their systems, which allows for quicker weight loss from exercising, dieting, or simply reducing food intake. I've seen hypothyroid women who cannot lose weight even when they eat like birds and choose only healthy vegetables. When they eat any food beyond their starvation diets, they gain two or three pounds immediately. They become very frustrated, because they know they are doing everything right.

Feeling cold

Many of my female hypothyroid patients hate the cold. They hate winter. They hate snow. They have a hard time getting warm and staying warm.

I've joked that many of them seem reptilian. Of course they do not like the comparison, but then I explain, "You see, reptiles don't generate their own heat; they rely on absorbing heat from their environment. Consequently, they find a warm rock when they are cold." They seem to hate the comparison a little less when I ask them if they take hot showers during the day, snuggle up against a warm hubby, put their feet on the hot air register, or find themselves holding onto a coffee mug to warm up their hands. Once they can see the little reptile in them, they understand.

Low-thyroid patients will be the first persons to complain about how cold it is in the winter or in air conditioning and the first persons to be fanning themselves in the summer or in a fairly unventilated space with a lot of people. They seek out the perfect climate (not too hot, not too cold).

Lack of sweat

The poor regulation in hot weather has to do with the fact that hypothyroid patients tend to be bad at sweating. Some might see that as a benefit. Hey, no sweat, less body odor. Yeah. That's one way to look at it. However, your body needs to sweat so that there is moisture on your skin. Then when the air or wind hits that moisture, it takes heat away from your body by evaporation. The result is a cooling effect. This is why we become so cold when we go swimming and step out of the water into the wind.

Hypothyroid individuals—especially those who have been hypothyroid since they were young—are so bad at sweating that they are those amazing people who go out for a run in 80-degree weather and show no sweat marks on their shirt at the end. Heavy sweaters (like me) think this would be an advantage, because you could exercise without getting "gross." But unfortunately, those nonsweating people are more prone to succumbing to the heat and may even subconsciously avoid exercise because it makes them uncomfortable. Sweat is a good thing: it cools us down when we're hot, and sweating is one way that the body releases toxins.

Swelling

I'm not talking here about swollen lymph nodes or even a swollen thyroid; I'm talking about edema in the extremities (arms and legs). Hypothyroid people tend to accumulate fluid in their hands, lower legs, and feet. If you're not sure that's you, pull down your socks. How long do the sock striations stay embossed on your legs? If it's for more than a minute, you definitely have swelling issues.

Any time that a gland in the body is incapable of doing the volume of work that is being required of it, the gland will swell. Swollen tonsils and adenoids are good examples of this. They are immune protectors full of white blood cells that are designed to make antibodies to help us fight infections. Small and unobtrusive under normal conditions, tonsils and adenoids grow and swell when they are fighting a massive infection or when they have become inherently too weak to do the normal amount of work. (Just a side note: from what I've seen in my office, most of the time immune assistance is being required of the tonsils because of food allergies and sensitivities. If the patient eliminates wheat or whatever allergen is active, the tonsils will begin to shrink on their own, with no further intervention. We can't always shrink them back down to normal size once the glands have swollen to five to ten times their normal size, but some shrinkage is guaranteed once the person's tonsils stop having to fight day and night against food allergens.)

When people's swollen tonsils and adenoids become too big, they can be removed surgically. And while, yes, anybody can live without their tonsils or adenoids, I prefer to keep surgery as a last resort. Why not pay attention to the symptoms and try to discover the cause so you can address it? I believe that God gave me my tonsils (as well as all of my body parts and functions) to me to help me live life to the fullest. I believe that they are part of His perfect plan. If I start cutting out parts because I can survive without them, then I cut out the potential that God put within me to help me to overcome obstacles so that I can live the best possible life.

Like your tonsils and adenoids, other organs and glands, such as your liver, spleen, and lymph nodes, grow swollen when they have been asked to do more work than they should. In the same way, your thyroid gland also swells in reaction to being overstressed. Because of the location of your thyroid gland in the front of your throat, this swelling can be visible as a protrusion in your neck, and this swelling is known by a familiar name: goiter.

As you may already know, a goiter results from an iodine deficiency. Because thyroid hormone is composed of such a large proportion of iodine, the gland cannot function properly without receiving regular amounts of iodine. Where do our bodies obtain the iodine they need? From the foods we eat. Iodine salts are concentrated in water, especially seawater, and they become available to our bodies through the eating of fish, seaweed, or crops grown in soil that has been enriched with iodine by having been underwater in centuries gone by.

Years ago, in the midwestern states of the United States and other regions that lack iodine-rich seacoasts, people used to have a hard time getting enough iodine. Quite possibly, when the glaciers came through the Midwest in ancient times, they scraped off the iodine-rich soil that had been left behind from the time when seas covered much of North America. Consequently, as midwesterners ate only food that had been grown locally, they gradually became deficient in iodine.

Goiters were often the result—swollen thyroid glands working hard to keep metabolism normal and perform other essential functions, but without enough iodine. Once the salt companies in the United States began to put iodine into their salt in an effort to make sure that Americans had enough of it, the number of goiters in the nation went down dramatically. Goiters remain a significant problem in other iodine-poor parts of the world, however.

Despite the fact that goiters are down in this country, I contend that hypothyroidism remains epidemic. Let me give you an example. Let's say you have a car factory in your town, but it is not making many cars. You might say, "Hey, I can help!" And you would then go out and buy hundreds of tires and radios. "OK," you'd say as you deliver the tires and radios to the factory, "now you can make your cars." While it's true that they may be able to manufacture more cars now than they could before, the truth is, they undoubtedly had other needs besides the tires and radios. They needed steel for the frames and glass for the windshields, and the list goes on and on. Plus, what about the workers? Are they being paid enough? Are they being taken care of?

In the case of hypothyroidism in America, we've solved the iodine issue for most people. However, other raw materials may be needed in order to make thyroid hormone.

Also, I believe that we are contending with a bunch of chemicals that inhibit proper thyroid function, essentially poisoning the thyroid gland and impairing proper communication between the thyroid hormones and the thyroid receptor sites in the cells of the body.

What Does Hypothyroidism Look Like?

What symptoms of hypothyroidism do I look for with my patients? As you read through the following descriptions, remember that you may have a hypothyroid problem without having all of these symptoms present in your life.

Poor healing

Many patients come to me for chiropractic care, but they can't seem to get better or stay better. The cells of their bodies cannot seem to keep up with the requirements of ordinary living.

Each cell in our bodies needs to be replaced. Cells along the linings of our lungs and gastrointestinal tract last only a few weeks, while the cells of our bones need to be replaced only every five to seven years. But all cells age and need to be replaced. The thyroid stimulates this routine turnover of tissue, and it also makes possible the healing the damaged tissues.

Let me give you a "for instance": Many patients report to me how wonderful they feel with exercise. They tell me that exercise gives them energy. With abundant physical exercise, they wake up more easily in the morning and feel energetic throughout the day. When I ask why they are currently not exercising if it has helped them so much, they always say the same thing: the pain stopped them. Where did that pain come from?

To explain that, I need to explain exercise to you. When I am weight training, the first goal of a starter program is figuring out what weight to start at. If I start too high, what happens? I will be *very* sore the next day. If I start too low, the exercise does me little or no good. When I initiate weight training, I'm notifying my muscles that I am not satisfied with their current ability and strength and that I want them to be able to do more. When I lift just slightly more than I am easily able to lift, some of my muscles experience damage as a result. Taking notice of the damage, my body tags the damage with inflammation (swelling and pain). My body has a mechanism (involving the thyroid) to heal that muscle fiber, this time making it stronger. (By the way, the body does the exact same thing with bone, which is why the experts always tell us to do weight-bearing exercise so that our hips and spines develop a higher density of bone tissue.) Once the current weight seems too easy, I increase the weights in order to set up this cycle again. I want my body to increase the capability of the muscle fiber to handle more weight.

Hypothyroid individuals feel so well after exercise because the act of exercising produces heat. As I mentioned earlier, a hypothyroid person does not generate enough body heat. So when they exercise, their bodies warm up, all their enzymes (that were stunted before by the lack of heat) begin to work properly, and they feel good— until the pain sets in. Their body's healing ability is challenged more than average by all of the lifting, running, or whatever type of exercise they have chosen to do.

A normal person can work out again two days after doing it initially and be ready for the next challenge. For a hypothyroid person, two days isn't nearly enough time to heal. Instead of developing strength, they end up adding damage on top of damage, (adding insult to injury). After a certain number of sequential workouts, they find themselves unable to proceed. Their pain overrides their desire to work out.

And of course, once they have refrained from exercising long enough to heal, their body temperature has returned to its "normal" low level, their fatigue has set back in, and now they have another excuse to not exercise. Not only have they lost any muscle progress they attained a few weeks or months ago, but also now they find that they are too tired to do the bare essentials—much too tired to start up an ambitious workout program again.

In other words, with or without workout regimens, low thyroid people suffer from chronic pains because their bodies are less capable of healing and self-repair.

Unhealthy hair, skin, and nails

Some of the most common symptoms of an underachieving thyroid (and, honestly, typically the easiest to fix) are dry skin; weak fingernails that crack, break, and peel easily; and hair that falls out easily.

Dry skin is easy to spot. Do you feel as though you constantly need to keep applying lotions to your skin? Or do you—like one male patient of mine—have unusual calluses that you didn't used to have? This patient came to my office with only two symptoms: fatigue and an odd callous formation on his hands that looked as though he worked as a professional tug-of-war player. He was a construction worker, but his job did not require an unusual repetitive motion that could account for the callus formation. Almost as an afterthought (because he wasn't cold and he was definitely on the thin side), I started him on Thyrosol.[2]

Within a mere two weeks, the extremely thick calluses on both of his hands were completely gone. He stopped taking Thyrosol then, because he thought he was completely better—and his calluses and fatigue returned. After that, he resumed taking the supplement for another six months, at which point he could stop taking it safely. The low thyroid symptoms did not return.

I see other dry skin issues very often with hypothyroid patients. One condition, follicular hyperkeratosis, is a skin condition characterized by excessive development of keratin in hair follicles. If you google it for images, you will see rough, elevated red bumps (sometimes with pus). This has been called *phrynoderma*. "Phrynoderma is a form of follicular hyperkeratosis that is associated with nutritional deficiencies. It is endemic to poor populations but is rare in developed countries. The term 'phrynoderma' was coined…in 1933 to describe the 'toad-like' appearance of the skin of undernourished labourers. This form of dermatosis can be caused by isolated deficiencies of vitamins A, B complex, C and E."[3] Remember this; you'll read more about the vitamin A deficiency later on.

Adult and teenage acne is very common with hypothyroidism patients. I suspect it has to do with the body's impaired recuperative powers and a deficiency of vitamin A.

One of the most common problems I see with female hypothyroid patients is their inability to grow strong nails. Nails that break, crack, or peel easily are a classic symptom of hypothyroidism. I realize that many of you have had this problem for so long that you do not even know it's a problem. If you can peel one layer of your nail off of another layer of your nail, you may be hypothyroid. If you can bend your nail back, you may be hypothyroid. If your nails tear, if they do not click when you use nail clippers, if you are unable to grow them to any reasonable length because of their inherent weakness, you may be hypothyroid. (I feel as if this is the physician version of Jeff Foxworthy's "You know you're a redneck, if..." jokes.) There are a great many reasons why someone can have weak nails, but if you combine this symptom with others, it's probably because you're hypothyroid. The good news is that the nails grow back fairly early in the treatment process once we start getting the thyroid up to where it should be.

Regarding thinning hair, I find that women especially can tell me the status of their hair if I describe it. (This hair loss is entirely different than what men experience with male pattern baldness or even receding hairlines.) I ask the following questions:

- Do you find a lot of hair in the drain after your shower?

- Do you often find yourself often cleaning excess hair out of your hairbrush?

- Do you feel like your hair is thinning?

- Do you find your hair all over the place?

- Do you find yourself wishing you had a collie like Lassie that you could blame because of all the hair on your black coat?

Women, please note (and men too, when male pattern baldness is not the culprit)—if your hair is thinning, this symptom is begging for your attention. Just like the nails, once the thyroid starts running properly, you should see more hair staying on your head and less departing. Also, one of the telltale signs of hypothyroidism is the loss of the outside third to one-half of the eyebrows. It might sound like an odd or unusual symptom, but I've seen it in a fairly high percentage of hypothyroid patients I treat.

Dry body syndrome

OK. I just made this name up. There's no such disease as DBS. But it is true that people with underactive thyroids never seem to have enough water (and oil) in them. I am unsure as to why the bodies of hypothyroid sufferers have this symptom, but I certainly see it often.

Besides having dry skin as I described above, their mouths are dry, and so are their eyes and their hair. Healthy skin and hair need their natural oils. To compensate for this lack, people who struggle with thyroid function have to make sure they use conditioner on their hair, and they probably feel their skin is like a sponge when it comes to lotion. When they apply lotion, their skin just sucks it up and they have to apply more. I ask my hypothyroid patients about their lotion use at home and I'm amazed at how much they go through.

Normally your body secretes oil through the pores of your skin and scalp. Oily secretions protect you from the outside world, and this same oiliness keeps the water that is so essential to your health body from evaporating. Women with long hair have been taught to brush their hair a hundred times daily to help transport their natural oil from their follicles all the way down to the tips of their hair.

When you become dehydrated or that oily protective surface is missing, your hair will dry out and become more brittle and prone to split ends. Your skin will feel dry, tight, itchy, and flaky. Hypothyroid individuals seem to retain insufficient water in the cells of their bodies, and, in the words of the Pepto-Bismol tag line, they fail to have enough oils in their body to "coat, soothe, and protect."

Routinely the eyes of my low thyroid patients seem to be dry or red or burning. Their mouths and lips are dry. Their "low water problem" may also explain why they are more prone to constipation. Natural bowel movements require sufficient water in the colon. That's why people who are prone to constipation are told to eat plenty of insoluble fiber, stop eating any foods to which they have sensitivities, *and* to make sure they are drinking plenty of water. But with a person whose constipation stems from low thyroid function, these measures will help only to a degree.

Blood pressure and heart disease

In the short term, your blood pressure and heart rate could theoretically go up with thyroid treatment, but eventually, as your body repairs itself, your mineral levels improve, and your body starts to handle stress better, you should find your blood pressure going down. This is the party line with regard to hypertension and hypothyroidism. However, if the hypothyroid body struggles with healing and properly replacing old tissue with new tissue, wouldn't the same thing hold true with regard to the heart and whole cardiovascular system? A 2008 Norwegian study followed twenty-five thousand people and noted a significant increase in coronary artery disease (which causes heart attacks) as TSH levels increased above 1.4.[4] The crazy thing about that is that the normal range for TSH is 0.3–5.0 for most labs in the country. Can you see that we're missing a bunch of people with problems?

In a study described in the May 2007 issue of the *Journal of Clinical Epidemiology and Metabolism*, one hundred patients who had essentially normal thyroid blood panels were studied over only twelve weeks of treatment with a synthetic thyroidlike hormone. Their total cholesterol and LDL cholesterol decreased, hip-to-waist ratio improved, study participants experienced less fatigue, and they lost weight. This was a study of patients taking thyroid help whose lab tests were normal for hypothyroidism![5]

Can we agree that hypothyroidism and heart disease are strongly related? I've quoted two studies, but there are at least a dozen that show a link.

Difficulty swallowing

Dysphagia is the fancy medical term for difficulty swallowing. This is a functional problem (not chemical) with regard to hypothyroidism.

When a person's thyroid swells, sometimes it swells out, and the person has a very visible neck swelling, as I described above (goiter). Other times the thyroid swells inward. In that case, due to its proximity to the esophagus (food pipe) and trachea (windpipe), it can produce trouble swallowing. A person can feel as if something is blocking food going down the esophagus or actually feel as if something has gotten stuck in there or keeps pressing in on the throat. Because the trachea can be involved, a person can also feel as if there is something in the windpipe that needs to be expelled by coughing it out.

I recently had a teenage patient who had a chronic dry cough (without producing any mucus). Theorizing that the cough stemmed from hypothyroidism, I provided some nutrients for the teen's thyroid gland, and, believe it or not, the swelling went down and the cough ceased within only a few hours.

Symptoms of Hypothyroidism at a Glance

+ Fatigue, exhaustion, low energy (even after twelve hours of sleep)

+ Weakness

+ Intolerance to cold

+ Dry skin

+ Dry and brittle hair, nails, etc.

+ Hair loss

+ Dry eyes and mouth

+ Weight gain, inability to lose

+ Inexplicably calloused skin on hands and feet

+ Edema of extremities

+ Chronic pain, muscle and joint aches

+ Lump in throat (hard to swallow)

+ Heart disease symptoms

+ High cholesterol

* Blood pressure problems
* PMS and menstrual cycle irregularities (prolonged and heavy)
* Infertility
* Yeast infections
* Poor healing
* Depression
* Chronic constipation
* Vitamin A deficiency
* Gallbladder dysfunction
* Acne (juvenile or adult)
* Thinning of outside part of eyebrows
* No sweat or almost no sweat
* Slow reflexes
* Decreased memory and concentration
* Low sex drive
* Anemia tendency
* Uterine fibroids
* Enlarged thyroid gland

Depression

Depression as well as other psychological conditions can be the result of adrenal issues, nutrient depletion, or fatigue. Any and all of these can be traced to hypothyroidism.

The ongoing challenge we have in treating hypothyroid patients is the amount of change that is necessary in order to develop a person's body (and emotions) working at a higher-functioning level. Depressive symptoms are definitely improved when we treat the whole person instead of just manipulating the body's neurotransmitter levels through antidepressants.

Fertility

I've had several hypothyroid patients who were helped to become pregnant by my treatments. (Side note: After more than ten years in practice, I have learned to rephrase my patient success stories so that none of them begin with lines such as, "I was instrumental in getting Julie pregnant." My initial attempts at storytelling led to some cocked eyebrows.)

The aspects of treatment that prove most helpful are:

1. Balance estrogen levels (See Appendix C for products I recommend to do this.)

2. Increase progesterone levels

3. Address and fix hypothyroidism

4. Perform chiropractic adjustments on lower back and pelvis

One challenging decision is whether to correct the low thyroid problem with a supplement or to give progesterone. I typically recommend a supplement, further recommending that the patient continue to take that supplement or something similar throughout her pregnancy. I've seen too many miscarriages when patients stopped taking the supplement when they got pregnant. Either they felt they no longer needed it, or their OB-GYNs convinced them that it wasn't a good idea.

I believe that if a woman needs a supplement to help her body become pregnant, she should probably stay on that supplement until her body can sustain the pregnancy on its own—which might be for the duration of the pregnancy.

Edema

What is edema? It's basically extracellular (not in cells or blood vessels) fluid that has leaked out from cells or blood vessels and has now accumulated in the tissues, otherwise called swelling. Myxedema is the type of edema that is most commonly seen in thyroid disorders.

It's pretty easy to see if you are edemic. The bones in your feet are no longer visible. Your extremities look puffy. You can see the striations left on your legs for several minutes after you take off your socks. Depending upon how tight your socks are, you might also notice a ridge where the top of the sock was. The stretchy fibers of your socks have pushed the fluid in the tissues under your skin out of the way.

Without using the sock test, you can test this on your own. Take your finger and find your shinbone. Half the way between your foot and your knee, push your finger down into your skin until you hit the bone. (This might be a bit painful if you are prone to chronic pain.) Hold your finger there for a count of fifteen seconds, and then let go. Do you see a dent? If you have edema in your leg, you will be able to both see the dent and feel it. And you will likely carry this dent over your shin for the next five to ten minutes as the fluid that you pushed out of that area takes a while to redistribute itself.

Other Reasons for Edema

Of course, there can be a number of reasons why people may have extra fluid in their upper and lower extremities and even their face. While avoiding the "death bed" explanations, here are some of them:

- ✦ *Toxicity.* I don't mean "poisoned" here. I mean that your body has waste products or toxins that have accumulated in your tissues. Back in the sixties and seventies when we dumped our waste into the Great Lakes or into our oceans, we thought dilution was the solution to pollution. Your body follows this solution when it will not allow water to leave your circulatory system and cells in order to dilute toxins that are present. The result is an increase in interstitial fluid (the fluid that surrounds your cells, keeping them moist), creating a large accumulation of extracellular (outside the cell) fluid, otherwise known as edema.

* *Protein deficiency.* A body with a dramatic deficiency in proteins will have a hard time making albumin. Albumin (yes, it is the main protein in egg whites) is the primary protein in the bloodstream, and it is responsible for maintaining the proper colloid osmotic pressure (COP). Albumin attracts water, causing more water to stay in the bloodstream. Without the albumin, the fluid seeps out of the vessels, causing edema or swelling. Such a swelling in the abdominal area (also called peritoneal cavity) is known as ascites (uh-SIGHT-ees).

* *Liver damage.* Since the liver is the organ that makes albumin, liver damage can lead to ascites.

* *Congestive heart failure and high blood pressure medications.* High blood pressure (antihypertensive) medications typically work by causing the heart to pump less hard. When the heart stops pumping as hard as it should, the circulatory system loses the healthy "back pressure" that keeps the blood moving through the capillaries and veins. After a while, the blood will have a hard time returning from a person's extremities. As a result, the fluid will start leaking out into the surrounding tissues, causing swelling.

* *As for congestive heart failure,* the right side of the heart is having difficulty pumping blood into the lungs to receive oxygen. The result is that side of the heart starts to fail, and the blood backs up from there and into the rest of the veins throughout the body, which invariably results in a blood "traffic jam," forcing fluid to find its way into the tissues and causing edema.

- ✦ *Situational.* Extended travel (sitting) or prolonged standing can induce swelling in the legs. Elevating the lower extremities will solve this type of swelling.

- ✦ *Pregnancy.* Pregnant women definitely experience swelling in their legs and sometimes hands. Some of that is due to the pressure of the baby against the veins carrying blood from the legs. Oftentimes pregnancy swelling can be an indicator of a protein deficiency (which is part of the condition called pre-eclampsia and eclampsia).

Vitamin A deficiency

One of the deficiencies seen with hypothyroidism is a vitamin A deficiency. Normally, your body takes the orange-colored beta-carotene from carrots and similar vegetables and converts it to the bioactive version of vitamin A with the help of your thyroid hormone. Some low-thyroid people can start to show orange hair and skin when they eat a large amount of orange vegetables such as carrots because the excess beta-carotene remains unconverted, so it builds up. Vitamin A is considered to be important for night vision, good skin, and viral infection protection; it also helps protect the body's mucous membranes from infections.

Gallbladder dysfunction

The gallbladder stores the bile created by the liver. Another problem seen quite often in patients with low-functioning thyroids is biliary stasis. The basic diagnostic premise of biliary stasis is that the bile in these patients has become thick and sludgy. Unfortunately this can rarely be confirmed by ultrasound (although it is possible to visualize gallstones and chronic moderate-to-severe gallbladder inflammation, which causes wall thickening) or cholangiogram (a functional test that is supposed to show blockages and bile flow).

Gallbladder dysfunction can be suspected in conjunction with some or even all of the following symptoms:

* Reflux

* Chronic right shoulder pain

* Chronic right upper back pain

* Chronic right-sided neck pains

* Intolerance to deep-fried, fatty, or greasy foods

* Chronic bloating or gas

* Periodic unexplained diarrhea or loose stools

* Pain over the right upper quadrant of the abdomen just under the rib cage

* Deficiency or difficulty in supplementing with fats such as fish oil or fat-soluble vitamins (vitamin A, vitamin D, vitamin E, and vitamin K)

Why do we often see gallbladder dysfunction along with hypothyroidism? It's hard to say. But I've seen it way too often not to link the two.

Biliary stasis worsens as a result of eating processed carbohydrates such as sugar, high-fructose corn syrup, and white flour (processed from wheat).

Yeast overgrowth

Yeast overgrowth often seems to accompany a low-functioning thyroid. I can't tell you which causes which. My gut instincts tell me that the thyroid problem, which causes low metabolism, low oxygen, acidic environments, and more, causes the yeast overgrowth and not the other way around.

Yeasts tend to grow more prominently in women with high estrogens (i.e., from pregnancy, estrogen replacement therapy, or birth control pills), in acidic environments, and wherever tissue oxygen is low. Sometimes a diagnosis of dysbiosis (a term made from "dys-" and "symbiosis") can be made, and dysbiosis of the bowel seems to correlate with hypothyroidism. Dysbiosis indicates an overgrowth in the intestines of pathogens such as yeast, harmful bacteria, viruses, or parasites.

Yeast is ubiquitous (meaning that types of yeast are everywhere). Everyone always has some yeast in the colon, but the aerobic (oxygen-loving) flora of the colon should be primarily *Escherichia coli* (*E. coli*), *Lactobacillus*, and *Bifidobacterium*. There are others, but most of them (*bacteroides, clostridium,* etc.) are anaerobic (which means they are unable to live in the presence of oxygen).

I like to describe your intestines as a backyard. Let's say you like to keep your yard green by mixing a few different types of grass. Nobody would consider it a badly maintained yard if, say in the late spring, one or maybe two dandelions popped up. It would still look green overall, and I would call that a fantastic yard.

However, different situations can cause some die-off of the grass, and then your yard becomes unsightly. Here in my part of the Midwest, we use salt in the winter to melt the snow and ice. We also go through times where it doesn't rain much. Environmental conditions such as these can lead to some die-off of the good grass species, causing the lawn to thin out or even show patches of dirt. (In comparison, such a thing might happen in your intestinal tract after a round of antibiotics. Many of the normal flora of the intestinal tract are killed off, leaving less-populated spots.)

Since weeds do better than grass in low-water regions, and they grow more quickly, it doesn't take much die-off to allow the crabgrass, clover, thistles, and more dandelions to take over. (This would be comparable to a yeast overgrowth in your gut.)

Symptoms of Yeast Overgrowth

Yeast overgrowth (typically intestinal) is diagnosed by either using an organic acid (urine) panel or by observation of signs and symptoms such as the following:

- *Skin yeast outbreaks.* These include ringworm, athlete's foot, jock itch, vaginal itching, and red areas of skin in areas where there is skin on skin (such as armpits and skin folds) or in areas where synthetic materials (underwear latex, for example) do not allow the skin to "breathe" as well. Yeast likes warm, moist areas.

- *Chronic chapped lips.* I typically refer to this as a Kool-Aid mustache in kids, and often it is indicative of yeast overgrowth. The kid licks his lips, the yeast gets on the skin and multiplies there (it's a warm, moist areas), and then it dries, leaving inflammation. It feels better when it's moister, so the child licks his or her lips again, adding more yeast to the area. The cycle keeps up until the area is treated/protected and the internal yeast overgrowth is halted.

- *Vaginal yeast infections.* These are possibly the best-known examples of yeast overgrowth.

- *ADD and ADHD.* While not a symptom of yeast overgrowth per se, ADD and ADHD as well as generalized "brain fog" can be exacerbated by yeast infections.

- *Sugar cravings.* The yeast thrives on sugar. Sugar cravings that are very difficult to resist can be symptomatic of yeast overgrowth.

- *Diaper rash.* Almost always, diaper rash is a yeast manifestation.

- *Excess flatulence.* Intestinal bloating can be due to excess intestinal yeast.

Back to the lawn analogy: to restore your lawn to its thick grassy state, you need to use a herbicide (a poison specific to the weeds) and reseeding. Weed and seed. In the case of yeast overgrowth in my patients, I do not bring out the big guns to kill all of the yeast (although there are prescriptions out there that can do that). I use natural compounds that slowly but surely change the patient's system to create an environment that the yeast does not care for. This use of supplements may take longer, but it also means having significantly fewer side effects. I also strongly suggest that patients cut back on all sugars (table sugar, high-fructose corn syrup, and even fruit and fruit-based foods) in order to starve the yeast. That's my "herbicide" phase.

Some people believe that the "seeding" should come with its own fertilizer too. A few doctors use an ingredient called FOS (fructooligosaccharide) that the normal flora like to eat. But I haven't found the need to do that. My patients seem to respond very well to providing the right mix of probiotics, which is what I consider my "seeding."

Like a grassy lawn, the thicker the normal flora, the less chance that the yeast will be able to reestablish a stronghold in the colon.

Fibromyalgia

Some practitioners theorize that fibromyalgia (and the equally hard-to-diagnose chronic fatigue syndrome) represents a collection of symptoms that can be traced to underlying hypothyroidism.

People speculate about whether or not fibromyalgia is a true disease. Truthfully, fibromyalgia is not a good diagnosis. It's a syndrome, which means it is an accumulation of a variety of signs and symptoms, all of which can come from a variety of causes. For instance, dry mouth is a common symptom of hypothyroidism (as well as other disorders), and we find it listed as a common symptom of fibromyalgia.

Fibromyalgia doesn't cause things. Fibromyalgia isn't a primary condition that arises from a certain organ, tissue, antibody, or even microorganism.

As a diagnostic term, fibromyalgia has allowed many people who have suffered from chronic pain to have a name for their problem. Forty years ago, these people were often called hypochondriacs or complainers since doctors could find nothing systemic wrong with them. But we still have no lab tests to diagnosis fibromyalgia. There are still no "go to" drugs that are used to treat fibromyalgia.

Medical doctors treat fibromyalgia by giving sleep aids for the insomnia, NSAIDs for the inflammation, painkillers for the pain, Synthroid for the hypothyroidism, and so on. They treat each individual sign or symptom of the condition.

I tell people that I'll give them the label if they want it, or we can just go after the primary issues that I find. A discussion of fibromyalgia is pertinent to a discussion of hypothyroidism, since that's commonly my end diagnosis. I start my diagnosis and treatment with an examination of food allergies and sensitivities. Next I "cut to the chase" and treat them for hypothyroidism. I may go after hormonal and adrenal issues too, if they are bad.

Dr. John C. Lowe, director of research for the Fibromyalgia Research Foundation, has concluded that, for many people, the fibromyalgia syndrome is a symptom of an underlying thyroid problem, not necessarily a disease unto itself. According to Mary Shomon, health activist on thyroid issues:

> [Dr. Lowe] feels that the typical patient's fibromyalgia is actually evidence of too little thyroid hormone regulation of certain tissues. According to Dr. Lowe: "…when I refer to fibromyalgia, I'm referring to a certain set of symptoms and signs of too little thyroid hormone regulation of tissues."[6]

This is speculative, but it makes sense. It's consistent with what we know. We know that hypothyroidism patients commonly have chronic pain, are tired all the time, do not heal well from injuries, and so forth. I think that a huge number of fibromyalgia patients could stand to have their thyroid function boosted, along with having their food allergies and sensitivities remedied, their adrenal/stress issues dealt with, and more—all pretty much what I'm doing here in this book.

Shomon goes on to explain:

When patients are already diagnosed as hypothyroid, [Dr. Lowe] is not surprised when they start to manifest fibromyalgia-like symptoms, such as various muscular aches and pains and difficulty sleeping. Dr. Lowe believes that, when someone has been hypothyroid, over time: "Hypometabolism imposes a lifestyle that can further complicate the hypothyroidism. For example, the hypothyroid patient may not be able to engage in enough physical activity to maintain normal muscle mass. Metabolic status is critically dependent on muscle mass; the lower an individual's muscle mass, the lower her metabolic rate."[7]

As you have read through the variety of symptoms in this chapter, did one or more of them "ring a bell" inside? Keep reading the following chapters to find out more about what to do if you think you have an underactive thyroid.

Chapter 6

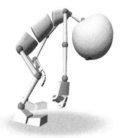

HOW MUCH THYROID HORMONE IS TOO MUCH?

I f some is good, more is better."

This may apply to many things, but it's not true when you're talking about thyroid hormone. Too much thyroid hormone causes a condition known as hyperthyroidism. A hyperthyroid person has too much thyroid hormone circulating in his or her system. The thyroid gland is going crazy making and secreting too much thyroid hormone for the body to use.

Unlike heart attacks, which can show their first symptom as death, hyperthyroidism makes itself known in time to do something about it. The symptoms of hyperthyroidism are very obvious and disturbing. For the most part, hyperthyroid people feel as though they have drunk way too much coffee or taken too many diet pills. People can have heart fluttering and palpitations, a rapid heart rate, trembling hands, diarrhea, sweating, insomnia, and excessive weight loss. Most commonly, I hear the complaint from hyperthyroid patients: "I feel like I'm crawling out of my skin."

Thyroid "Thermostat"

People suffering from an overactive thyroid gland have such a highly stoked inner furnace that they require a ton of fuel (food). Imagine if you had a thermostat on your fireplace and your job was to keep that fireplace to maintain that thermostat at a certain level. It would be fine as long as you had a cord of precut wood ready to go out in back and you had scheduled regular deliveries of more wood to keep the fire fueled. But eventually you could run out. Then, as the fuel dwindled, your task would become a high-pressure one.

You would run outside to fetch another load of wood and discover an empty wood rack. Now what? You would run down into your basement where you would break apart your wooden shelving unit for fuel, figuring you could get along without it. Next, though, you would have to choose between your coffee table and your dining room chairs. The situation would escalate. At first you would limit yourself to wood products only, but eventually you would burn anything that would catch on fire, including plastic, expensive items like your laptop, and even your clothes. Eventually you would start to demolish parts of your house to keep up. Before long, you would no longer have a house at all, just a smoldering fireplace.

The same thing can happen to a person's body with hyperthyroidism. First the body will burn through the stored carbohydrates and the fat stores. Eventually, needing more, it will start burning muscle. Because the excess thyroid hormone circulates throughout the body, symptoms appear throughout the body and are almost too numerous to list. With time, most of them can become quite serious—life threatening if you do nothing about them.

In addition to severe weight loss and usually an increased appetite, other symptoms that may appear along the way can include the following: muscle wasting, hyperactivity, inability to tolerate heat, loss of hair, aching muscles, muscle weakness, an apathetic attitude, fatigue, irritability and anxiety, possible mental impairment, hypoglycemia, tremors and jerking limbs, heavy sweating, increased urine production along with excessive thirst, atrial fibrillation of the heart and an accompanying shortness of breath, loss of sex drive, nausea and vomiting, and a cessation of the menstrual cycle in women. Often a person's eyes peer at you with a kind of bug-eyed "stare," sometimes but not always related to a hyperthyroid condition known as Graves' disease. (More about that just below.)

Graves' disease

This is the best-known type of hyperthyroidism, because it is the most common and because of some well-known people who have received this diagnosis, such as Barbara Bush. In spite of its relative rate of recurrence, Graves' disease often goes undetected for years because so many of its symptoms are so "ordinary" and/or easily attributed to other causes.

Graves' disease is an autoimmune disease (a disease in which a person's body creates antibodies against itself), and it seems to run in families. Because its cause is not clearly understood, the treatment consists of reducing the excess thyroid hormone by various means in an attempt to return the body to a more normal level of function.

Thyroiditis

As you can tell from the "-itis" suffix of the word, thyroiditis means an inflammation of the thyroid gland. The two primary types of inflammation are known as Hashimoto's thyroiditis (which is also an autoimmune disease) and De Quervain's thyroiditis (also known as subacute thyroiditis and easily confused with an unrelated thumb condition named for the same person). Both Hashimoto's thyroiditis and De Quervain's thyroiditis are hypothyroid (low thyroid) conditions that may initially appear as a hyperthyroid disorder.

Postpartum thyroiditis

Postpartum thyroiditis, known as PT for short, afflicts about 7 percent of women during the first year after they give birth. Like traditional thyroiditis, it starts out as hyperthyroidism. After a few weeks or months, it can revert back to normal or dive into hypothyroidism. This can be quite disconcerting and confusing for the new mom.

Thyroid storm

Aptly named and very serious, this is a rare but life-threatening, emergency condition resulting from a literal "storm" of thyroid hormone. Patients must be hospitalized, resuscitated, and treated (if they survive) in a manner suited to the initial cause.

Symptoms of a thyroid storm, also known as thyrotoxic crisis, can include a high fever (as much as 107°F), rapid pulse, diarrhea, irregular heartbeat, and extreme weakness to the point of coma. A number of factors can cause a thyroid storm, including ingesting too much hypothyroid medication or supplementation and abruptly stopping drugs that were pushing down excess thyroid hormone in patients with hyperthyroidism.

Symptoms of Hyperthyroidism at a Glance

- Hyperactivity, nervousness, restlessness
- Insomnia
- Anxiety, irritability
- Trembling
- Goiter or thyroid nodules
- Fatigue
- Diarrhea or irritable bowel
- Increased appetite
- Increased thirst
- Increased sweating
- Increased urine output
- Weight loss
- Inability to tolerate heat

- Rapid/fluttering heartbeat
- Amenorrhea or irregular periods
- Muscle weakness, aches
- Mental impairment
- Exophthalmos (bulging eyes)
- Chronic cough
- Itchy skin

Diagnosing Hyperthyroidism

Hyperthyroidism will show up on a blood workup. For that reason you need to have your blood drawn to confirm the diagnosis.

If the blood test shows that you do have hyperthyroidism, you need to direct the next question to yourself: are you doing this to yourself? Assess your diet and any supplements you may be taking. Are you on prescription thyroid medications? If so, maybe it's possible that you need less. (If that's the case, your medical doctor who prescribed the medications will help you cut back.) Have you taken excess iodine supplements, kelp, or seaweed? Are you dosing yourself with high amounts of L-tyrosine? If so, just stop. Once you discontinue using the products or eating the iodine-bearing foods, your system should settle back down to normal.

If your assessment does not turn up anything suspicious or if reducing your intake of possible troublemakers does not work, you will need to consider your next step carefully. Hyperthyroidism is often treated by doses of radioactive iodine or by surgical means. The surgery is called a thyroidectomy, and it means a complete or partial removal of the thyroid gland. It goes without saying that a thyroidectomy is irreversible. You may prefer to start with less-invasive treatments, especially if you can tolerate your symptoms a little longer.

You will be advised that, after destroying your overactive thyroid gland, you can replace your missing thyroid hormone artificially with a prescription preparation. However, no prescription thyroid replacement can ever equal your own natural thyroid hormone. That's why it is best to try first to balance the production of your own thyroid hormone before trying anything more drastic. You can always have your gland irradiated or removed, but you can't go back and adopt the more conservative approach after you've been too aggressive.

Always remember this rule of thumb: start with the least harmful procedure and proceed to the most aggressive as a last resort after trying everything else first. I consider herbs, nutrition, chiropractic massage, physical therapy, acupuncture, reflexology, magnets, and homeopathic treatments to be good first-resort treatment options because most of them have a very short list of things that can go wrong. With any of them, usually the worst thing you can do is to waste some money and time. But any adverse reactions to the above treatment options are minimal and *reversible*. Needless to say, it is far more difficult if not impossible to reverse the effects of surgery complications or radiation treatments.

What do I suggest for a natural remedy? Although it can be a bit tricky to get the dosage perfect, the herbs lemon balm, motherwort, and bugleweed can often prove to be very effective at helping to get your thyroid back to normal. Along with that, I always work with individuals nutritionally, both to build up the person's strength and to remove any possible sources of internal stress.

What Should a Hyperthyroid Patient Do?

Many patients have walked into my office with overt hyperthyroidism. One woman's condition was so bad that she said the medical doctors who were managing her case wouldn't even attempt surgery or irradiation. She was shaky, sweating, unable to experience any decent amount of sleep, and losing incredible amounts of weight. Her thyroid levels were off the charts.

We found that supplementing her with bugleweed (one of the herbs I mentioned above that is known to help with hyperthyroid problems) several times a day calmed down her thyroid. In the meantime, we helped make sure that she got restored nutritionally, and we also rejuvenated her adrenals. Pretty soon we were able to wean her off the bugleweed. Almost miraculously, her thyroid gland had returned to normal.

Other patients have thyroid nodules, which they have been told should be removed surgically because they are considered precancerous. While it's true that the nodules can become cancerous later, I do not feel that a thyroidectomy or irradiation should be the first step in medical treatment for hyperthyroidism, in particular because it represents fear-based advice.

Now it's true that if you have polyps in your colon—and it's well known that such polyps can eventually become cancerous—it's a good idea to remove them during a colonoscopy. Then they can be tested to see if they are already cancerous, and in any case they will no longer remain a danger to the individual. But notice that the doctors do not immediately suggest the complete removal of one's entire colon as soon as they see one polyp.

Why is this different from the thyroid gland? One reason is obvious—nobody has made a drug or an artificial colon that can replace the one they would take out. While thyroid hormone replacements do exist, in my opinion they are never as effective as a person's natural thyroid hormone, and I disagree with the medical establishment's opinion that thyroidectomy and subsequent prescriptive treatment is the safest and most satisfactory option for treatment.

If people have been exposed to nuclear radiation, as is happening, as I write this book, with the Japanese people near the Fukushima Daiichi Nuclear Power Station, which was damaged in the March 2011 earthquake and subsequent tsunami, they do stand a greater risk of developing cancer. That's the reason why people near sites with dangerous radiation try to take normal iodine (usually in

Lugol's solution or high-potency Iodoral, a brand name of potassium iodide tablets) to saturate their thyroid with normal iodine in an effort to make it less likely for their thyroid to pick up the radioactive iodine. Even so, effectiveness is difficult to determine, since often the people who have been exposed to radiation do not develop cancer for as long as forty years.

Thyroid nodules are like micro-goiters. If only some sections of the thyroid gland are inflamed, the result is going to be local hypertrophy or swelling of only some of the tissue, which will appear to be a small protrusion or bulge or nodule. As with other thyroid problems, the preferred first line of attack with thyroid nodules should be giving the thyroid everything it needs in order to function the way it is supposed to, not surgical removal. (See chapter 9 for a full discussion of treatment options.)

If, however, the nodules have already become cancerous, surgery or irradiation to destroy the nodules is the only good option. As the patient, I would always ask to see my cytology report to make sure that cancer cells have been found—and that surgery or irradiation will take out only as much of the thyroid gland as is absolutely necessary. If I can keep some healthy tissue, I want to do that.

Regarding treatment by irradiation of the thyroid gland, I have a further concern. The thyroid gland, however, does not distinguish between radioactive iodine and nonradioactive iodine. When the thyroid gland picks up radioactive iodine in the course of medical irradiation of the thyroid, the thyroid gland undergoes radiation exposure. I don't know about you, but I want to minimize my exposure to harmful radiation, even if it's in the name of health and healing.

Hyperthyroidism is something to be concerned about. However, in some cases the condition will simply resolve itself without intervention. That is why I am so adamant about putting off the surgical or radioactive iodine options for as long as possible. Once you destroy your thyroid gland, you cannot grow or transplant a new one!

The obvious exception to trying noninvasive options is if your life is in jeopardy. Nobody chooses a natural, healthy, long-term approach during a heart attack or when you've had a gunshot wound. Be smart about what is truly a life-threatening emergency requiring aggressive intervention and what conditions will allow you the time to take a more conservative approach to treating your hyperthyroid condition.

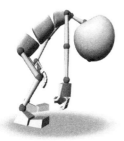

Chapter 7

WHAT HORMONES AND SUBSTANCES INHIBIT YOUR THYROID?

As you begin to explore the possibility that your collection of symptoms may point to thyroid dysfunction—or even if your physical and emotional problems turn out to result from a different cause—the last thing you need to contend with is a known stressor. In this chapter we will take a look at some common substances that can "intimidate" the healthy functioning of your thyroid gland.

Most of them are natural substances; some turn out to be your own hormones. They create problems when they get out of whack for some reason—or when, as in the case of water-purifying additives, your body becomes exposed to too much of some substance such as chlorine.

Food Allergies and Sensitivities

As I told you in chapter 4, "Healthy Eating," some people believe that gluten can impair thyroid function. I'm not convinced of that across the board. I certainly do not think I need to keep grains away from people who have normal functioning thyroid glands.

However, a lot of people have issues with specific grains or grains in general or dairy or sugar and high-fructose corn syrup. In my experience, these can play a role in impairing normal thyroid function. In the autoimmune condition called Hashimoto's thyroiditis, food allergies and sensitivities can exacerbate the autoimmune response.

"Autoimmune" implies that your immune system has been confused and considers some part of your own body, such as your thyroid, to be an enemy that must be destroyed. Your body begins to make antibodies against whatever seems to be the invader. Antibodies are proteins that "tag" the invaders so that the other parts of the immune system (reticuloendothelial system, or RES) can find them and finish the "removal" of the invader. When your body crosses the line into autoimmunity, it has been making antibodies that cross-react with the associated body part because they appear to be similar to a true invader.

The first step in overcoming any autoimmune disease is to find out any pertinent allergies and sensitivities and to completely remove those substances from your diet or environment.

It doesn't work to try to limit or reduce the amount of a substance you ingest or become exposed to, because even if you consume the allergenic substance once every few days, that consumption can act like a booster shot. You know what a booster shot does. When people receive a vaccination, they often end up having a series of injections in an effort to increase their antibody level against the organism targeted by the vaccination. The first shot allows the body to "see" the organism and produce a relatively small immune reaction (similar to getting the first bee sting). The second and subsequent booster shots boost antibody production. In essence, by getting the series of injections, we are trying to remind the immune system not to become lazy with regard to this organism but rather to keep watch against it, attacking it whenever it detects the harmful organism.

In much the same way, our bodies can remain in attack mode as, through repeated exposure, we "remind" our immune systems to react against otherwise harmless foods or substances that have been once tagged as invaders. If this happens on top of other formerly healthy body functions that have been compromised in any way, such as occurs with thyroid dysfunction, the negative effects pile up more quickly and recovery gets bogged down.

Chlorine and Fluorine

Again referring back to chapter 4 about choosing foods and beverages that are good for us, we need to take a long, hard look at our drinking water. If we don't, we may be compromising our health and our children's health on a daily basis.

Why? Because both chlorine and fluoride, chemical elements that are used in municipal water treatment facilities to sterilize our drinking water and to reduce cavities in teeth, are similar to bleach and therefore are toxic to our bodies. Specifically where your thyroid gland is concerned, you need to take a special look at these particular elements.

Since your body requires iodine to make thyroid hormone, and since iodine is considered a halogen (any of the five elements that form part of group 17 [IUPAC style periodic table, formerly VIIA] of the periodic table: fluorine, chlorine, bromine, iodine, and astatine), the thyroid gland is more apt to pick up fluorine and/or chlorine instead of iodine. And since fluorine and chlorine are poisons, the result is a sick thyroid gland that is unable to keep up with demand and make enough thyroid hormone.

Neither chlorine nor fluorine is required for health. In fact, both are considered human toxins. As a result, I and many others believe that they should either not be added to our water supply by municipalities in the first place, or they should be purified out of our water by a home purifier that is a distiller or a reverse-osmosis unit.

Just so we're all clear, let me add that I'd rather have chlorine in my water than live fecal bacteria. But I also believe that we should be looking into other forms of nonchemical water sterilization such as ozone, heat, ultraviolet, and more. The bottom line is simple:

adding chemicals to our water supply, which leaves chemical by-products in the water that you and I drink, is not a healthy idea.

Mercury

Mercury is a toxic heavy metal that is found in nature, but it is found in more concentrated forms as dental fillings (called silver-mercury amalgams) and thimerosal (mercury preservative used in all vaccinations for years up to just recently; it is gradually being removed and replaced with other preservatives).

A high percentage of Americans have amalgam fillings in their teeth. Especially as the fillings grow older, they begin to degrade and release mercury into the person's body where it is readily reabsorbed by the moist tissues of the mouth and digestive tract.

Mercury can also become a problem when people consume too much fish, because, from the water they live in, fish and shellfish concentrate mercury in their muscle tissue. Larger fish that are higher up the food chain inevitably have higher concentrations of mercury because they consume smaller fish—thus increasing their own mercury load by ingesting the entire burden of the mercury that the smaller fish was carrying.

Below is a list of fish with the highest amounts of mercury. The "FDA Average" column reports averages (in number of milligrams of mercury per 1 kilogram, or 2.2. pounds, of fish) calculated by the US Food and Drug Administration in its ongoing monitoring program launched in 1990. (ND stands for no data.)[1]

Species (Domestic Samples)	FDA Average	Atlantic Catch	Pacific Catch
Anchovies	0.04	ND	0.04
Cod	0.10	0.06	0.11
Crab	0.06	0.26	0.15
Flounder	0.05	0.08	0.07
Halibut	0.25	0.25	0.28
Herring	0.04	0.04	0.14

Species (Domestic Samples)	FDA Average	Atlantic Catch	Pacific Catch
Lobster	0.17	0.28	0.17
Mackerel	0.15	0.22	0.09
Mussels	ND	0.08	0.03
Oysters	ND	0.07	0.06
Perch (ocean)	ND	0.08	0.08
Pollock	0.06	0.02	0.06
Salmon (fresh)	0.01	0.13	0.04
Salmon (canned)	0.05	ND	0.04
Scallops	0.05	0.01	0.04
Shark	0.99	0.75	0.80
Shrimp	ND	0.04	0.03
Snapper	0.19	0.28	0.25
Swordfish	0.98	0.98	0.98
Tilefish	1.45	1.45	ND
Tuna (fresh or frozen)	0.38	0.28	0.24
Tuna, albacore (all forms)	ND–0.76	0.47	0.17
Tuna, yellowfin (all forms)	ND–0.76	0.31	0.06

From whatever source, when your body takes in mercury, it recognizes it as a toxin and stores it away in sites such as the thyroid gland in order to remove it from doing immediate damage in the bloodstream. Unfortunately, especially where your thyroid gland is concerned, this means that mercury competes, on the enzyme level, for the mineral receptor sites within the cells of the gland. As a result, needed enzymes get a "busy signal" when they begin to stimulate the production of T4 and T3 hormones, thus impairing the manufacture of fresh thyroid hormone.

Once people started realizing the danger of mercury toxicity, they began to ask their dentists to replace their old amalgam fillings. And even though eating fish provides a great source of iodine, which is good for the thyroid, people have had to balance that against the harmful effects of a higher intake of mercury. The thyroid gland is in the middle, just trying to do its job in spite of the substances that interfere with its healthy functioning.

See chapter 9 to read about how the mineral selenium can help rid your body of excess mercury.

Goitrogenic Foods

I need to address goitrogenic foods because they are believed to contribute to the creation of goiters, which, as you will remember, are swellings of the thyroid gland resulting from an iodine deficiency. *Goitrogenic* means simply goiter (goitro) creating (genic, as in "genesis").

Goitrogenic foods, at least in raw form, contain enzymes that inhibit iodine from being utilized by the thyroid gland. These vegetable foods, many of which are termed "cruciferous," such as cauliflower, broccoli, cabbage, and brussels sprouts, lose their fairly limited goitrogenic capabilities when they are well cooked.

Having said that, I have not seen any impairment of my patients' thyroid production from their consumption of goitrogenic foods, which are otherwise good for a person's health. Therefore I'm not recommending banishing these foods from your diet at all, especially since elimination of the goitrogenic enzyme requires cooking for at least thirty minutes, which will also destroy the good enzymes and vitamins.

My word to you is to *know* this information but not to restrict your vegetable consumption unless you feel that you continue struggling with hypothyroidism despite doing everything else first. We Americans eat far too few veggies anyway, and I certainly don't want to cause you to deny yourself something that is so good for your health just because a few people may have noticed the problem.

Soy

Controversy surrounds soy foods. On the one hand, soy can be used as a substitute for dairy products and animal protein, and it seems to carry phytoestrogen (estrogenlike) properties. In Asian cultures where a large amount of soy is part of the diet, many quantifiable health benefits seem to ensue, such as a lower rate of heart disease and fewer menopausal hot flashes for Japanese women compared to women in other cultures.

The well-known holistic practitioner Dr. Joseph Mercola has come out extensively against soy.[2] Some experts say that soy inhibits thyroid function. Thus, as a food it falls into the category of a goitrogen. I have not been able to refute or confirm the goitrogenic soy claims. However, based on my own clinical experiences, I do know that many of my patients who have had problems with dairy products eventually form allergies to soy products as well.

My own recommendation is to be aware of the possibility of soy-compromised thyroid function. The apparent positive benefit of soy in Asian cultures is more commonly associated with fermented/cultured soy (miso, tofu, etc.), so unless you are really struggling to balance your thyroid, I typically approve the use of these types of soy products a couple of times a week. Soy milk, soy ice cream, soy cheese, and soy flour are a different matter. There are much better flours out there. (See list in Appendix D.) As for milk, I strongly suggest either rice milk or (unsweetened) almond milk as a better alternative to soy milk. Unpasteurized (raw milk) cheese can be difficult to find, but I believe it produces less negative reaction than other kinds of cheese (pasteurized or soy). Besides, it takes so many ingredients to help soy to resemble real cheese. Take a look at an ingredient list sometime. As you know, I try to avoid overprocessed foods because they introduce so many variables into my patients' diets.

Estrogen

Speaking of estrogen, let's delve a little more deeply into the subject. While it may seem like a sidetrack to talk about the "female hormone," I do not consider it a side issue in view of the fact that so many of my thyroid patients are women.

As I mentioned earlier, most women experience changes in their metabolism during pregnancy and upon delivery. During pregnancy, thyroid hormone function can be inhibited by increased estrogen. After delivery, postpartum thyroiditis can manifest as either hypothyroidism or as hyperthyroidism. Sometimes, as I mentioned earlier in the book, it can manifest first as hyperthyroidism and then switch to hypothyroidism. Endocrinologists can diagnose the problem, but of course it would be overkill to assault an overactive thyroid gland with surgery or irradiation, or to treat an underactive thyroid with artificial hormone. I prefer to support a woman's thyroid gland using nutrition and natural compounds and herbs until the thyroid hormone production self-regulates.

More importantly, women should be aware of how many of their physical and emotional struggles relate to estrogen and its counterpart hormones—and how these symptoms can overlap with overactive or underactive thyroid hormone issues.

When I say "estrogen," I am referring to three types of estrogen: estrone (E1), estradiol (E2), and estriol (E3). Along with progesterone, these comprise the female hormones.

Estrogen and progesterone have many opposing functions in a woman's body. As you can see below, similar symptoms identify estrogen excess as well as progesterone deficiency:[3]

Estrogen Deficiency

- Dry skin
- Headaches
- Hot flashes

- Night Sweats
- Sleep disturbances
- Vaginal dryness/atrophy
- Heart palpitations
- Depression
- Yeast infections

Estrogen Excess

- Water retention
- Craving for sweets
- Nervousness, anxiety, irritability
- Heavy irregular menses
- Fatigue
- Weight gain
- Mood swings
- Low thyroid symptoms

Progesterone Excess

- Weight gain
- Headaches
- Anxiety
- Mood swings
- Irregular menses
- Depression
- Infertility
- Fuzzy thinking
- Acne

Keeping in mind also the "fright/fight/flight" mechanism, which kicks in when the body feels stress from a hormonal source as well as from advancing wild animals, we see more overlapping symptoms:[4]

Low Cortisol

+ Fatigue
+ Allergies
+ Cravings for sweets
+ Irritability
+ Chemical sensitivities
+ Symptoms of hypothyroidism
+ Symptoms of low progesterone

High Cortisol

+ Same symptoms as low cortisol
+ Bone loss
+ Anxiety
+ Sleep disturbances
+ Depression
+ Low libido
+ Hair loss
+ Anxiety
+ Elevated triglycerides

The dysfunctional elevations of cortisol and estrogen mess up a woman's system. It is my further contention that menopausal hormone replacement therapy further interferes with normal estrogen levels. As it was originally delivered, the replacement estrogen came from pregnant horse (mare) urine, thus the name Premarin, and it contained only two (estradiol and estrone) of the three estrogens. The missing estrogen (estriol) happens to be considered the one that has the most protective effect against cancer. Premarin also contains equilins (horse estrogens). Since God did not make human bodies to handle the waste hormonal metabolites that are specific to horses, it was no great surprise to those of us on the natural side of health care when the National Institute of Health (NIH) halted its large-scale Women's Health Initiative involving thousands of women in 2002 because the adverse reactions (significantly increased risk of strokes, heart attacks, clots/embolisms, as well as breast cancer) in patients taking Premarin and PremPro were so alarming.[5]

Hardly ever are studies of this magnitude stopped so abruptly. But in this case, the participating women were told to stop taking Premarin and Prempro, which is Premarin given in conjunction with a synthetic progesteronelike preparation called progestin.

My point here is that I strongly believe we should not be extending hormones for women after their bodies reach the point (based on God's original plan) that they don't need so much of those hormones anymore. Just look at the bad results. However, if a woman has a low production for her age, I do not see any reason why not to help her make more or to prescribe bioidentical hormones (available at compounding pharmacies) to boost her up to where she needs to be.

As with other hormones, we get into trouble when we try to achieve more youthful results than we should. Guys who take anabolic steroids (basically excess testosterone) to become stronger can get into trouble from doing it. Human growth hormone is considered by some to be the medication version of the "fountain of youth," but taking more than what would normally be produced at your age (we always make some growth hormone even after we're done growing) is going to be hard on some of your organs. Prednisone, a very powerful anti-inflammatory medication, a miracle drug for some people, is basically cortisol (made by the body's stress gland), and yet its negative side effects are legion. Taking prednisone is like having the fire department spray a million gallons of water into your house for a small stove fire. Yes, it does get rid of the fire and keep it from spreading. However, the peripheral damage is so extensive that it likely outweighs the benefits. Couldn't the benefits have been obtained with a more conservative, less aggressive approach?

In the same way, we should only be giving estrogen and progesterone if someone's body seems to be deficient. As you can see from this closing chart, hormones affect each other, so any consideration of thyroid hormone levels must take the interrelationships into account.

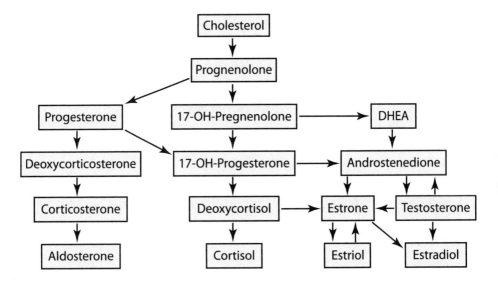

All of the above hormones look very similar. They are all considered steroids, and the base from which all of them are made is cholesterol. You can imagine that if stress hormones are being secreted and produced in high amounts, the person's body would likely shunt production to the adrenal side and lack enough of the raw material to make the sex hormones. The result? Women under stress will quite often lose their menstrual cycle. Men under stress have impotence issues as well as often a lower desire for sex.

How does all of this related to thyroid? Excessive amounts of circulating estrogen are known to inhibit the conversion of T4 to the more active T3. So does too much cortisol.

Cortisol (also referred to as hydrocortisone and part of the class of steroids called corticosteroids) is controversial. You could read something online or in a book and decide, "I need to find a medical doctor to prescribe hydrocortisone for me." (Many times on blogs and forums people will abbreviate hydrocortisone to HC.) But is HC really what we need?

The idea behind providing it is this safety net concept we spoke about when we were discussing stress in the third chapter. Think of the body as the cartoon character Linus and the adrenal glands as his security blanket. Most of the time, Linus's blanket has no purpose. He just carries it around wherever he goes. Occasionally he uses it for what it was designed for: to cover himself to stay warm. However, most of the time it's just there to make him feel secure. (I know, at the end of *A Charlie Brown Christmas* he uses it as a Christmas tree wrap...but I have no wonderful adrenal comparison for Linus's selfless use of his blanket in that case. Oh well, no analogy is perfect.)

My point is this: our bodies are the same with regard to the adrenals. With the adrenals there, our bodies can feel safe. Our bodies know that if push comes to shove, the adrenal glands are ready and capable to keep the body safe. Confidence in that "security blanket" allows all of the body systems to function the way they were designed to.

People are getting HC, and it appears to be helping them. However, what will happen if we keep going down this road? Why supply the hormone that your body should be producing and secreting on its own?

Although I am not a specialist in pharmacology, I can see that HC appears to be a short-acting, more bioidentical version of cortisol, compared to prednisone, which is a longer-acting, synthetic version of cortisol. Prednisone comes with the equivalent of its own chapter in the Physician's Desk Reference (PDR), which gives information about all the different prescriptions available, both benefits and side effects. It is well known that excess cortisol in the body impairs and inhibits the thyroid from functioning properly. For that reason I would steer clear of using any prescription that appears to try and do what cortisol does.

Remember, when the body secretes cortisol, it shifts the body into the sympathetic mode, which changes the body's priorities. Healing, maintenance, and repair are no longer high on the priority list. That's not the result you want to achieve when you add extra cortisol to the mix!

The take-home message here is this: Whether we refer to the adrenals glands as a security blanket, a bucket that we need to keep filled, or an emergency fund that we need to stop making withdrawals from, we need to put a sign on it that says, "FOR EMERGENCIES ONLY." Stress messes with you. Focus on fixing problems that are depleting your adrenals (chronic viral infections, food allergies/sensitivities, worry, etc.) and actively seek to find supplements that support your adrenals. The result? Your body will function much, much better.

You weren't made to be stressed beyond periodic, short bursts of time. Always remember that. A healthy life is designed to be lived at peace.

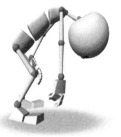

Chapter 8

TESTS TO DIAGNOSE THYROID PROBLEMS

Before I became a chiropractor, I was a medical technologist. My first college degree was a bachelor of science in medical technology, a four-year degree in laboratory medicine. We learned how to draw blood and run laboratory tests and how to recognize blood cells, bacteria, and parasites under the microscope. We studied all the diseases of blood cells. We learned about infections that are common and infections that are rare. We became skilled at distinguishing different viruses, species of bacteria, types of fungal infections, and parasitic infestations. We gained knowledge about cholesterol and blood sugar. We were taught which diseases could be diagnosed with a simple urine specimen and which with a blood test.

I know. Too much information, right? But most of us don't think about who runs those tests or the training they have had. Someone needs to run these tests. Before I became a chiropractor, that someone was me.

Like me, a great many chiropractors obtain advanced specialty degrees in sports medicine, neurology, orthopedics, pediatrics, and radiology. My specialty is in nutrition and internal medicine. My training in laboratory medicine gives me an extra tool in my diagnostic tool belt.

After I draw someone's blood in my office, I spend a good forty minutes with the patient at a subsequent appointment going over the results of the lab tests. As a physician, I consider it one of my roles not only to give the patient the correct remedy or advice, but also to explain why. I need to explain what will possibly happen if we just leave things alone. I need to tell the person what we can do to correct a problem. My patients are comforted by the fact that I will be redrawing their blood and rerunning the tests to see how the treatment is working.

How to Use Blood Tests

Most blood tests are pretty straightforward. Unless an individual is on medication that interferes with test results, a blood test will not show elevated blood sugar (glucose) if a person is not diabetic. Likewise, people can't be anemic unless the blood work actually shows a reduced number of red blood cells. Blood test results are that clear-cut.

When it comes to the thyroid gland, it can be a bit trickier. Back in chapter 5, I introduced you to a hormone called TSH (thyroid-stimulating hormone). TSH is secreted by the pituitary gland in response to TRH (thyrotropin-releasing hormone), which is released by the hypothalamus to encourage the thyroid gland to increase production and secretion of T4 (thyroxine). The test for TSH was initially developed in 1973.

The idea behind the test is that in many cases of hypothyroidism, the pituitary's release of TSH to stimulate the thyroid works about as well as a boss yelling at an employee to work harder. Then the boss goes from a yell to a scream, and some employees respond to this type of motivation. So do some thyroids. Typically, though, despite the pituitary "screaming in the thyroid's ear," the thyroid gland cannot produce enough thyroxine. The thyroid is still under-achieving despite the elevated levels of TSH. What that amounts to is this: if the TSH is elevated (unless some obscure pituitary tumor is present), then hypothyroidism is also present.

What if the pituitary is sluggish and lazy? The TSH will be low to normal. Then if the hypothalamus starts telling the pituitary that the body needs more thyroid hormone, it's just too bad. In other words, even though it would seem that testing for TSH levels would prove whether or not a person's thyroid hormone levels are normal, it does not—because other factors can be involved.

Perhaps an analogy might help. Running a TSH test would be the equivalent of checking the bank account of an insurance salesman in order to determine his effectiveness as a salesman. On the surface, it seems like an effective way to assess his job skills. The better the salesman, the more money in the bank, right? However, mitigating circumstances will surely skew those test results. What if his wife works? If so, their bank account could reflect her income. What if they are currently on a spending spree? This would certainly drain their account, and it could appear that he does not earn much, if any, money. What if he is delinquent in paying his bills? His account may look extraordinarily good in that case, but only because he has not paid out what he owes to people.

Do you see what I'm saying here? Proper medical standards of care consider TSH a great screening tool to assess a patient for hypothyroidism. However, there are too many variables. What's the health of the pituitary? What's the health of the hypothalamus? We might see plenty of T4, but is there enough T3? And finally, are the hormones communicating normally with the cell receptor sites? Because it looks only at a single facet of the complicated workings of the thyroid system, the TSH turns out not to be such a good screening test after all. Let me explain why.

Screening tests

In theory, screening tests shouldn't omit anyone who has the condition/disease. Granted, you might catch some people who don't have the condition in your net because of how broadly you throw it, but the plan of a thyroid-screening test is to miss as few hypothyroid patients as possible. Once you catch all of the true positives, as well as some false positives, then you need to use a more sensitive method for screening through all of these patients in order to toss out the false positives (the people who don't have hypothyroidism) from the results.

Confirmatory tests

Once you catch all (and then some) of the hypothyroid patients by screening, you should then perform confirmatory tests. To make a good diagnosis, you need a test that has what's called "high specificity." Simply put, you want to make sure that everyone who gets the diagnosis actually has the disease.

With the confirmatory test, we do not want any false positives, and this matters the most when diagnosing certain conditions. For instance, you don't want to tell a woman that she's pregnant until you're sure. You do not want to diagnose pancreatic cancer (a cancer with a very poor prognosis) unless it's true.

I explain all of this because that's why I consider the TSH to be a terrible screening test. It leaves a bunch of people out. How do I know? Because every week I see people who are looking for answers after their doctor informed them that their thyroid is functioning just fine. Little did they realize, when they wandered down the street to me, that I would end up treating their thyroid glands—and that they would get better as a result.

Now, critics will say, "Of course, if you rev up the metabolism of someone who is fatigued, they will enjoy more energy, and it proves nothing about the thyroid." But if I give thyroid help to people whose thyroids are normal, we can tell right away. Either they will experience no change, or they will go into hyperthyroidism. But if they were experiencing low thyroid function after all, we will be able to assess their hypothyroid symptoms (which include far more symptoms than just those involving energy levels) and see how they've been helped.

Simply put, if I give help and it helps, I helped them. Done. Regardless of the results of that initial blood test.

How Can Blood Tests Lie?

It's true that we have very little to go on if we can't rely on blood tests. I'm not saying blood tests are junk. Blood tests are reliable for diagnosing anemia, diabetes, cholesterol levels, as well as many other conditions.

But we can't rely on the blood test to tell us *everything*, especially in some situations. When you become sick, your body responds. A good doctor can spot-check your symptoms and figure out a likely diagnosis from a physical exam and a personal history. In my physical diagnosis class in chiropractic college, we were taught that about 95 percent of the diagnoses will be made by the time we're done with the history.

Of course I use physical examinations, along with lab tests and X-rays, to confirm what I think, but a good doctor knows which questions to ask and how to differentiate between two conditions that have similarities. Much of the work lies in asking the right questions.

You might say, "Well, sure, but that was chiropractic college, and you didn't have to do what medical doctors do." And yet we did have courses in pathology, microbiology, laboratory medicine, geriatrics, pediatrics, endocrinology, and so forth to equip us so that if we ended up in a rural area that lacked doctors, people could come to us for a reliable diagnosis. Most chiropractors do not use all this knowledge on a regular basis because most of them are treating patients for back pain and headaches. However, it doesn't mean they aren't trained in diagnosing a wider spectrum of diseases.

Taking a good history and doing a proper exam are lost arts. We rely too much on our high-tech (and high-expense) equipment and not enough on our experience and intuition as doctors. Not everyone with a headache needs an MRI.

Introduction to
Thyroid Lab Tests

A beginner's guide to thyroid lab tests must include the following ones. Most of them have some uses, but I have indicated my opinion of their degrees of usefulness.

Remember, lab test ranges tend to be created by statistics, using the standard statistical Gaussian curve:

Serum Calcium (lab)

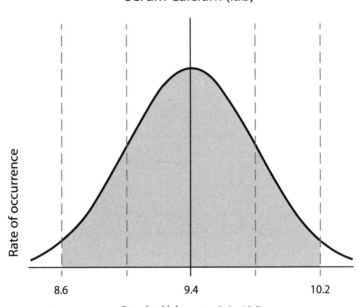

Standard lab range: 8.6 - 10.2

Typical values will be calculated from the compiled results of lab tests. "Mean" indicates the average. It hits the peak of the bell curve because the apex of the curve implies that that lab value was seen the most often. "SD" means standard deviation. All of the middle region from –2 SD to +2SD encompasses the middle 80 percent of all of the lab values. Many times labs take the middle 80 percent and call it the "normal" range.

I have two problems with that: (1) the blood test values come from the sick people who are tested at hospitals and doctor's offices—unlikely places to find a preponderance of healthy people, and (2) just because lab statistics show up in the middle 80 percent, why should that indicate that the middle 80 percent of our society is healthy? If we took, say, the middle 80 percent of all of the six-foot-tall American males based on weight, that range (probably between 190 and 270 pounds) does not necessarily represent a healthy range, although it definitely represents an accurate American distribution.

Serum Calcium (optimal)

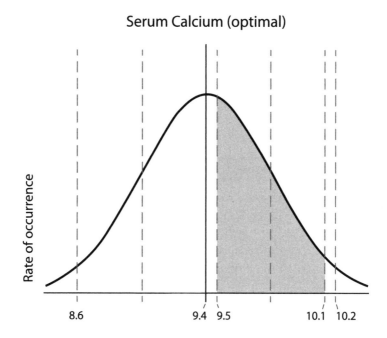

Dr. Berglund's optimal lab rage: 9.5 - 10.1

In the second graph above, we look at what most labs have determined to be "normal," or, as we referred to above, the middle 80 percent based on the average. The normal calcium range goes from 8.6–10.2. However, if I have a patient who has a "low-normal" calcium reading of 8.8, I'm pretty confident that person needs calcium supplementation.

In my office, I use "optimal ranges" that are typical for people who are healthy. I try to have my patients' test results fall within those ranges. In the above graph, you see how my range for calcium compares to the statistical "normal" ranges. I'm not saying that someone who comes in with a calcium of 9.1 is diseased, but my goal in treating patients is to find trends before they become diseases. I try to find deficiencies before the person's body is forced to compensate with a workaround in order to continue functioning.

The Tests

Traditional thyroid screening tests, some of them improvements upon older ones, include the following:

- ✦ **TSH.** The thyroid-stimulating hormone is released by the pituitary gland, and this test measures it. This test is believed by most medical professionals to be an adequate screen. Some have tried to make the TSH more relevant. They consider individuals to be hypothyroid if their TSH is less than 2.0. But that's not good enough, in my opinion. I believe that an elevated TSH (above 4 or 5) most likely indicates an underfunctioning thyroid gland. We have discussed this at length in chapter 5 and earlier in this chapter. Please do not use the TSH alone to tell you when your thyroid level is normal!

- ✦ **Free T4 (FT4).** Thyroxin (T4) is the hormone made by the thyroid gland. The "free" designation implies that it is not bound, which means that it has no carrier protein and therefore is in its active form. Test results: Hypothyroid if less than 0.7 (optimal range: 0.7–2.0).

- ✦ **Free T3 (FT3).** Triiodothyronine (T3) is more bioactive (some estimates have it at twenty times more active) than T4 is. Since this hormone is unbound, it is active. If you want to run blood work to see what your functional T3 levels are, this is the test to use. Test results: Hypothyroid if less than 2.3 (optimal range: 2.3–4.2).

✦ **Reverse T3 (rT3).** This hormone is made by the body in response to stress, when the body is trying to conserve energy, or during a serious illness or trauma. Excess T4 gets converted into rT3, which blocks the thyroid receptor binding sites from being acted on by active thyroid hormone. (This seems like a cruel hoax to someone who is hypothyroid, but the mechanism was set up to help.)

✦ **Anti-TPO.** Thyroid peroxidase antibodies give evidence that a person's body is amassing an immune attack against the thyroid gland—which is a bad thing. Many doctors do not consider this to be a very important test, but it tells us if the person's immune system is trying to destroy thyroid cells. It's important to deal with this issue first before we work to support the thyroid gland. (If I were a Southerner, I would say, "It makes more sense to kill the foxes in the chicken coop than to buy more chickens.")

✦ **Total T4.** This T4 test was more popular before the FT4 became available. However, since this test measures both bound (inactive) and unbound (active) T4 hormone, it doesn't tell us much. It doesn't make sense to find out how much inactive hormone is coursing through a person's bloodstream.

✦ **T3 Uptake (T3U).** T3U or T3 resin uptake (T3RU) is a percentage that is used to measure the capacity for T3 to be bound. Useless by itself, it is used primarily to measure the free thyroxine index (FTI), which is also called T7.

✦ **Free Thyroxine Index (FTI) or T7.** This is a calculation of the total T4 multiplied by the T3U percentage. This test was the lab standard measurement before TSH. It can be misleading, and I do not recommend using it.

What Are We Looking For?

The primary diagnoses within the hypothyroid category are as follows:

* Hypothyroidism

* Subclinical hypothyroidism

* Tissue resistance to thyroid hormone (TRTH)

* Peripheral thyroid hormone resistance

There are some rare conditions that I have not listed here, but honestly I have never seen them. Also, some of the above diagnoses (as far as maybe most medical doctors are concerned) are more hypothesis than diagnosis, but resistance diagnoses are the only real ways to describe and label these hypothyroid patients whom the lab tests show as "normal."

As far as blood work is concerned, many doctors make a diagnosis of hypothyroidism when the TSH is elevated above 3 or 4 or 5 (depending upon what lab and which practitioner you see). As you've heard many times from me, I may go ahead and treat a patient for a low-functioning thyroid even if the TSH is normal and even if the FT4 and FT3 numbers are looking good, if they have enough hypothyroid symptoms to justify going down this road.

Many other factors help contribute to the severity of hypothyroid symptoms. As you know from reading this far in the book, I consider it essential to take a detailed look at nutritional considerations. Because the following categories lend themselves to some form of testing, I have included them in this chapter about laboratory tests.

Iron and Hypothyroidism

Anemia is a condition that has known associations with hypothyroidism. Anemia is simply a reduction in the number of red blood cells in your blood stream, or a deficiency in their function. Red blood cells contain a substance called hemoglobin, which attracts oxygen. The primary function of blood cells is to carry oxygen from the lungs to the rest of the body. A deficiency of blood cells or anemia will therefore result in symptoms of low oxygen, which start initially as fatigue.

Some anemia is genetic (such as sickle-cell anemia or thalassemia). Others are due to defects in the liver or spleen. Still others are due to deficiencies in substances such as vitamin B_{12}, folic acid, copper, vitamin C, and iron, all of which are necessary to make healthy red blood cells.

Besides occurring due to impaired production of red blood cells, anemia can also occur from excessive blood loss. Women who bleed excessively during their periods can become anemic. People who take too much ibuprofen, naproxen, or aspirin can become anemic from gastrointestinal bleeds that occur as a side effect of this class of drugs (NSAIDs).

Iron is the active ingredient in hemoglobin. Most cases of blood loss or bad digestion deprive the body of the amount of iron it needs to make blood cells. Iron in the human body exists in several forms. It is carried around the system by a protein called transferrin, which is made in the liver. That is why, if a person's liver is going downhill, anemia will often be the result, even though adequate amounts of iron appear to be present. The person's body just cannot move it around.

Testing Iron Levels

How can we assess iron status? Most commonly, the following lab tests will be ordered:

+ **Serum Iron:** This is the amount of iron present in the liquid portion of the blood (not in the red blood cells).

- **Ferritin:** This is the iron that is stored in the body (backup supply). We can always tell how bad the deficiency is and how long it has been going on by looking at the level of storage iron.

- **Transferrin:** This is the body's carrier of iron in the bloodstream to deliver it to the spleen, liver, and bone marrow where it can be incorporated into red blood cells.

- **TIBC:** Total iron binding capacity is the percentage of transferrin that still could carry more iron if necessary.

- **CBC or complete blood count:** This looks at the number of red blood cells and white blood cells and how much hemoglobin is in each red blood cell.

- **Reticulocytes:** This is an old test, but it will look at how many of the red cells in the blood are young. What will happen in the body of someone with anemia is that the bone marrow will release blood cells before they are completely ready to be sent into circulation because some oxygen-carrying ability is better than none. This test can tell if the person's bone marrow is working at catching up but just has a lot of work to do, or if the red blood cell production is impaired.

Ferritin and the Thyroid

Doing some research for this book, I read an article posted on a website titled, "Ferritin, Iron and Hypothyroidism." It was written by Janie Bowthorpe, who has written a book called *Stop the Thyroid Madness* (the website goes by the same name). The article presents an interesting correlation: low ferritin and hypothyroidism. Since ferritin is a storage form of iron, I was intrigued as to why this might be. Certainly women who have low-functioning thyroid glands are known to have harsher menstrual periods than other women, and they have also been shown to have a lower-than-normal amount of stomach hydrochloric acid.

Being low in thyroid "can also lower your body temperature (common for those on T4-only thyroxine [prescription], as well) which causes you to make less red blood cells."[1] Once you become anemic, then you can develop "symptoms which mimic hypothyroid—depression, achiness, easy fatigue, weakness, faster heart rate, palpitations, loss of sex drive, hair loss and/or foggy thinking,"[2] which causes patients to think they are not taking enough thyroid medicine. If they therefore increase their dosage, they can end up with hyperthyroid symptoms.

Blowthorpe adds, "In turn, having low iron levels decreases deiodinase activity."[3] What does "deiodinase" mean? The prefix "de" always means to undo something (e.g., defrost, decode), "iodin" obviously refers to iodine, and "ase" is a suffix used strictly for enzymes. So what it means is that deiodinase is an enzyme that removes an iodine atom from the thyroid hormone. A T4 molecule with four iodine atoms attached to it will become T3, with three iodine atoms, if the deiodinase enzyme acts on the hormone. It seems that iron plays a role (along with other minerals) in this conversion of T4 to the more bioactive T3 hormone. In addition to this conversion, iron also seems to play a role in TSH production and T4 production. Thus, having low iron levels contributes to low thyroid hormone levels.[4]

For detailed information about what to do with test results, go to the next chapter and look for the section on treating anemia.

Allergy Testing

Because food allergies can definitely inhibit thyroid function and will add an unnecessary physical stressor on your system, I believe it to be critical to deal with food allergies. However, the word *allergy* will mean different things to different people in the health care field. Let me give you some background.

If you've been to an allergist, most likely your treatment has been entirely focused around finding allergies that cause redness, hives, swelling, coughing, sneezing, sinus congestion and nasal drainage, and sometimes anaphylaxis. Allergies with these symptoms are histamine-based allergies or IgE allergies. Most allergists who are medical specialists have been trained to focus on allergies that make histamine.

Types of Immunoglobulins

Immunoglobulins (antibodies) are abbreviated as Ig and include several different types: IgA, IgD, IgG, IgE, and IgM. The word *antibody* refers to a specific immunoglobulin that has been made to fight a particular foreign invader. Without making this into an immunology course, let's briefly discuss the types and their significance:

- **IgA** is an immunoglobulin that is found in the secretions of the mouth, nose, eyes, ears, digestive tract, and vagina. The secretions provide a barrier in those places as a person's body comes into contact with the outside environment.

- **IgD** is the least common antibody, and the least is known about it.

- **IgE** is the immunoglobulin that, when activated, causes a person's body to respond by releasing histamine from certain white blood cells that have histamine-containing granules. The result is usually hives.

- **IgG** is the most common immunoglobulin in the human body. It is in all bodily fluids. When people refer to antibodies, they are most likely referring to IgG. When individuals receive vaccinations or have infections, the body "remembers" the infection and for many years can continue to make specific antibodies (IgG) to that specific virus. Periodically, a person may receive a booster shot, which reminds the person's immune system to keep producing that antibody.

- **IgM** is a nonspecific immunoglobulin. It is the first to respond to an infection until the body can make enough IgG to take over. It's a macromolecule that is five times larger than the other immunoglobulins. It tends to stick together in colder temperatures (it's therefore called a cold agglutinin). The reason that's important to understand is because patients whose fingers or toes routinely turn white and then even bluish in response to cold (and sometimes stress) have a condition called Reynaud's phenomenon, which means that their stuck-together IgMs have blocked certain arterioles (small arteries). Their blood vessels vasoconstrict in response to stress, allowing less blood to flow into their hands, causing them to feel cold and causing the clumped IgM's to block the flow of blood. The result is a loss of the red hue.

The point of listing all these immunoglobulins in a sidebar is to tell you that a medical allergist will tend to run an IgE panel. It's fine to run an IgE panel, but most likely if you have the kinds of allergies/sensitivities that the IgE panel will detect, you can probably figure them out on your own. IgE allergies are considered type I hypersensitivity reactions, which means that they happen very soon after exposure (immediately to four hours). For that reason, most people can figure out what they were exposed to within the previous four hours that was unique or different than what they're used to: a cat, a dog, peanuts, some medication, pollen, hay, dust, and so forth. (The exception would be to tell a patient what specific type of pollen was bothering them; however, since I'm not treating airborne allergies, this information is not critical to my treatment of the thyroid.)

The more complete way to blood-test through the medical doctor is by using an IgG or (better yet) IgG_4 panel. The other four types of hypersensitivity reactions (types 2 through 5) are almost all IgG-based, which makes sense since IgG makes up 75–80 percent of the total immunoglobulins in the human body. With IgG reactions, the body may not start reacting until six hours post-exposure, and reactions could still be increasing up to seventy-two hours after the item initiates the body's response. Regarding food allergies and sensitivities, that means that by the time you eat your next meal and maybe even the meal after that, you are only starting to react to your first meal. This makes figuring out the sensitivity a huge challenge without the use of a more complete panel test.

Allergy or Sensitivity?

I need to clarify what I mean by "allergy" and "sensitivity." An allergy, as we discussed above, is a hyper-reaction by the immune system to a substance that should not be causing a reaction. My runny nose from a cold is not an allergy because my body is supposed to be fighting viruses. If I have a runny nose from cleaning my dusty basement, it may indicate a dust allergy, because dust should be inert or harmless to my body. I might need to cough to get the particles out of my nose or lungs, but it shouldn't be an ongoing response. With an allergy, my body confuses what is harmful with what isn't harmful. It loses track of what constitutes a foreign invasion versus simply a foreign substance. It's a discernment issue.

Sensitivity is a broader term. It means that something my body doesn't like causes a negative reaction in my body, whether it triggers an immune response or a nonimmune response. We say, "I'm sensitive to that." For instance, a diabetic is sensitive to sugar. One person may be sensitive to the mercury in amalgam fillings, and another may experience a reaction from drinking chlorinated water. None of those reactions are due to the memory response of the immune system, but they remain, nonetheless, sensitivities.

Testing for Allergies and Sensitivites

I have used two methods to figure out food allergies and sensitivities: lab tests and manual muscle-testing. Predominantly in my office, I use manual muscle-testing because I believe it provides me with more accurate testing than any lab tests that I have run. However, most providers do not use this method, probably because it appears to be less objective than a lab test.

A great many natural health care providers reliably use tests from the following companies to give accurate food testing results:

+ ALCAT test—The ALCAT test measures changes to a cell in response to exposure to a food or chemical, so the results go further than allergy testing (IgG or IgE) and measure intolerance/sensitivity. This makes it a more sensitive test than what would typically be run by most allergists or medical doctors.

+ Sage test—This company tests the blood for reactions to food. Because it is designed more as a cytotoxic test (looking at how the red blood cells react to foreign material), some find this test to be more comprehensive than a traditional IgG or IgG4 food allergy test for this reason.

+ ELISA/ACT test—Many allergy sufferers (if they've done enough Web surfing) have come across this test. As a test, this has been the "mother of all allergy testing" for years. The reason for that is the vast number of allergens that it tests for. Once you run the ELISA/ACT test, you really feel that you have left no stone unturned. But it's a very expensive test, and its blood processing is trickier than with other tests.

+ Genova Labs—This lab (formerly known as Great Smokies) does a wide spectrum of testing. Their food allergy testing is primarily IgG-based.

+ Metamatrix Labs—This lab also does a wide spectrum of tests. Their food allergy testing is also IgG-based. They are fairly inexpensive.

This is certainly not an all-inclusive list and, as the technology improves, other companies will find better ways to assess food allergies and sensitivities. I would recommend always going to a naturopath or DABCI board-certified chiropractor to have these tests evaluated.

Cholesterol and
Thyroid Function

If blood work shows that you have elevated levels of LDL ("bad") cholesterol, you may want to consider the cholesterol-thyroid function connection. By increasing your thyroid function, you can lower your cholesterol. In my office, I have been able to lower the cholesterol levels of many of my patients simply by improving the efficiency and output of their thyroid glands.

At times, providing hypothyroid supplementation to a patient causes the patient's system to go into overdrive (into hyperthyroidism or too much thyroid hormone). My first clue is usually the person's heart rate or reports of insomnia or feeling jittery or shaky as if overcaffeinated. However, if the patient does not have any of these obvious symptoms, I may decide that they have become hyperthyroid based on a blood test for cholesterol. Typically, test results for a hyperthyroid patient show a low cholesterol level (less than 140).

Now I know you're thinking that you have never heard of cholesterol being too low. However, low cholesterol can cause problems. It has been associated with major depression and increased suicidal tendencies. We also see low cholesterol levels in patients who are near the end of their lives and their livers are shutting down. It's called an "ominous sign" when cholesterol levels dip below 140, when combined with other signs and test results. (The other two reasons for low cholesterol besides "near death" that I've seen in my office are impaired gallbladder function—and excess thyroid hormone.)

Body Temperature Test
and Thyroid Function

Years ago a doctor named Broda Barnes figured out that a chronically low body temperature could help diagnosis a person with a low-functioning thyroid gland. Based on his discoveries, I have provided instructions and a convenient chart in Appendix A in the back of the book to help you record and evaluate your temperature over a period of days.

Your basal body temperature is your temperature when you first wake up in the morning. It is your basic or baseline body temperature. Once you start moving around, your muscles start burning fuel and producing heat as a by-product. So to capture your true basal temperature, you need to take it even before you get up to brush your teeth or go to the bathroom. You can purchase a special basal thermometer (available at drugstores), which will tell you your temperature to a tenth of a degree, or you can use an ordinary thermometer. Keep it on your nightstand next to your bed. Basal thermometers are very popular with women who are trying to become pregnant, because their temperature shifts at the time of monthly ovulation. Most basal thermometers come with a temperature-plotting chart. Make some extra copies of the chart that comes with your basal thermometer, or use the chart in Appendix A.

Take your temperature before you move about, either by mouth or by putting the thermometer in your armpit. Your armpit temperature is called your axillary temperature. Regardless of how you take it, this temperature reading should be your lowest of the day.

I know some of you are sitting there reading this, nodding and saying to yourself, "I really don't need to take my temperature. I'm always low, in the 96s and 97s." You might be surprised. A normal armpit temperature should be 97.5°F–98.2°F, and a normal oral (mouth) temperature should be 98.4°F–98.8°F. If it's true that your oral temperatures are consistently in the 96s and 97s, it's very likely, in my clinical opinion, that you are hypothyroid.

Take your temperature for four consecutive days. Even if you know that your temps run low, it's important to have a pretreatment baseline. Once you have a baseline based on several days in a row, you will be able to see how your baseline temperature rises as your system improves on treatment.

What? Where? How?

Some tests, such as the test for urine pH, blood pressure, and basal temperature, can be done in the privacy of your own home.

For most of the tests, though, you will need someone else to run the tests for you. It's easiest if you have a natural-oriented doctor who can do it (and they might even be covered on your insurance). Occasionally workplaces offer to provide a panel of blood tests and give you the results back. Someone recently told me that his insurance company was sponsoring a free blood test and that they would put an additional three hundred dollars into the HSA (health savings account) of whoever participated. This is obviously a good deal.

Online sites can provide you with blood tests if you send the sample to them yourself. All you have to do is have a lab draw your blood and spin it down, and then you can mail it in. However, you need to make sure that you have someone who can help you look at the results. If you can't find someone who can do that for you and you need the blood test analyzed, you can get in touch with my office. We usually do this via e-mail.

We all like lab tests. They are objective. It's hard to argue with a number. When I see the H (for high) or L (for low) on the blood test sheet, I know that no one will question my diagnosis. However, we need to be aware that lab tests only assist us to confirm what the patient's body is already telling us. When I'm stumped with a patient, I have no qualms about ordering a large panel. I admit it. I'm fishing. I pray, "God, show me what I'm missing here." With the results of a blood test in hand, I can see why the patient is anemic, if the kidneys or liver are struggling, and if the patient's blood sugar is creeping up too high.

Numbers do not lie. They might mislead us a bit as with TSH test, but they do not lie.

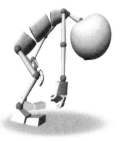

Chapter 9

RESURRECTING THE THYROID

When treating patients for low thyroid, all I do is provide the patient with the raw materials that their thyroid gland needs and proper stimulation if their thyroid has become lazy and—ta-da!—the thyroid starts to work properly again. Because I am not providing exogenous hormone (hormone that was made outside of the patient's body), but rather I am supporting the patient's own body to function on its own, their thyroid glands end up stronger. In contrast, if patients receive Levoxyl, Synthroid, or Armour (porcine thyroid), the hormone itself is being furnished from the outside, so the patient's thyroid gland doesn't need to recover the ability to manufacture its own hormone.

My approach to treatment matches the sensible adage: "Give a man a fish, and he eats for a day. Teach a man to fish, and he eats for a lifetime."

People Differ

Each one of us has things we do well and things we don't do well. Some of us are good at administration, and some of us are terrible at it (that's me, by the way). Some of us love speaking in front of crowds, and others hate it. (There is a study that shows some people are more afraid of public speaking than they are of death.)

Our bodies differ too. Some of us have trouble handling

inflammation. Some of us generate free radicals easily and don't have enough antioxidants to quench them. Some of us are prone to cancer. Some of us tend to gain weight. Some are predisposed to getting heart disease. Some of us are the first to become sick in our families; some of us never seem to catch the cold or flu that everyone is getting. Some people feel great after physical exercise, and others feel worse.

My job is to help you understand yourself better so you can tailor your approach to your own health. No advice fits all situations. Even when I give you good "rules of thumb," you may find that you don't fit the average pattern. For example, the standard advice when supplementing with calcium and magnesium is to take them in a 2:1 ratio. However, your gastrointestinal tract might be great at absorbing magnesium and yet terrible at calcium absorption. So why should you waste effort taking the magnesium if all you need is calcium?

Thyroid Prescriptions vs. Thyroid Supplements

Hear me very clearly here: I'm not opposed to people being on prescription thyroid hormone. Some people genuinely need it. Because I am not a medical doctor or a pharmacist or even a patient for whom thyroid hormones have been prescribed, I am unable to tell you to stop taking your medications. Did you hear that? Do not stop taking any of your medications just because my book talked about how great the natural approach is. My goal here is simply to present an overview of treatments for thyroid gland insufficiencies from my fairly extensive experience as a health care provider. You can find out more explicit information about prescription thyroid hormone from those who have been trained to provide it.

The most popular thyroid prescriptions are called Synthroid or Levoxyl (levothyroxine). As synthetic versions of T4 (thyroxine), they only remedy a T4 shortfall and do not address T3, and they are the least effective (from my observation) of the thyroid prescriptions.[1]

Most of the rest of the thyroid hormone prescriptions draw their thyroid hormone from the glandular tissue of porcine (pig) thyroid glands. The most popular and long-established one is Armour porcine thyroid, although new companies are coming into the game all the time. Recently, Armour has had some tangles with the FDA.

As I have said many times, I believe that people should start by seeking to help their own bodies to function without outside help. I strongly believe that we should restore normal body function first rather than sending in the troops to do the work that our bodies are not doing. Then, once we determine that our efforts have not enabled our bodies to return to normal functioning capacity by using nonsurgical and nonpharmaceutical approaches, we can explore the prescription options that are not restorative but rather substitutional.

Recommended Thyroid Supplements

In my treatment of hypothyroidism, I have settled on eleven different thyroid formulations that I carry in my office. I have listed these, together with their ingredients and some further comments, under Dr. B's Suggestions in Appendix C. (See Recommended Thyroid Supplements.) I choose from the following list, depending on what each patient needs:

- Thyro Complex
- Spectra 303T
- THY-O
- Thyroid-120
- Thyroid Plus drops
- T-100
- Thyrostim

- Medastim
- Thyrosol
- GTA
- GTA Forte
- GTA Forte II

You should be able to obtain these supplements from your nutritionally oriented health care provider or often directly through online sources. (See Where to Find Nutritionally Oriented Doctors in Appendix C.)

Take a Commonsense Approach

Please remember (as if I haven't stated it a hundred times already) that you are unique. My goal in writing this book is to empower you to take control of your decisions. I want to give you options for "translating" what your body is trying to tell you so you can treat it the way it wants you to. When I state a dosage or a range, you must understand that I'm not prescribing that for you, although you can "try it on for size." If you feel confused by the complicated information and all of the options for self-treatment, you'll need to find a good health coach to work with you and help you with your questions. It may take you a while to get a feel for what to do. Even as an experienced health coach, I am still experimenting with treatments in some very complicated cases.

The reason I devoted an entire chapter to healthy eating is that your first step should be to clean up your diet. Remember that wheat, soy, sugar, high-fructose corn syrup, and sometimes dairy can contribute to a low-functioning thyroid. You also need to remove the chlorine, fluorine, and heavy metals from your drinking water. This is important for you to know: if you don't want to change your diet or don't think that you can do it, I suggest you take a more pharmaceutical approach.

Supplements to
Support Thyroid Function

Most of the time I take a very hands-on approach to analyzing and assessing proper dosages with my patients. In the next few pages I will be going over the supplements that I give out at my office. Sometimes I will be quite adamant about sticking to the particular brand name that I am recommending. Believe me, it's not because I own stock in the companies that I recommend. If I recommend a certain product from a certain company, it's because I've tried similar products from other companies and gotten very little to no results. I want to keep you from making the mistakes I have already made.

The simple fact is that there are bad brands out there. When you find a generic drugstore or discount store version of a supplement, please assume it's no good until proven otherwise. To find out which brands are better, ask someone who works at the health food store. If you already know which brands are good, you can seek them out on one of the good vitamin stores online.[2]

I follow a few general rules when I treat patients for hypothyroidism. First, I don't start supplementation until the patient has started improving his or her diet and stress tolerance. Second, because the thyroid increases a person's metabolism and therefore energy, I recommend taking any thyroid preparations in the morning and at lunch—not at night when the patient needs to sleep.

Also, because my approach does not provide hormones but rather raw materials and general thyroid support, we really don't know how much is going to be enough. For that reason, I start patients out on one tablet or capsule in the morning, with food, and one at lunch, with food. For a minimum of two days I ask the patient to watch for any good results, and also to allow for their bodies to indicate that it's too much.

"Too much" means they are experiencing hyperthyroid symptoms—heart palpitations or an increased heart rate, feeling jittery and shaky, or even just seeing your hand tremble when you hold it in front of you. "Too much" is always a bad thing, but it's not an emergency. Typically these unpleasant symptoms will last anywhere from minutes to a couple of hours. In the literally thousands of thyroid cases that I have treated, I have only seen someone's body continue to stay excessively elevated two times, and those times were eventually brought down by bugleweed. Since you may be trying to treat yourself here, it may be a good idea to buy some bugleweed ahead of time. (I recommend a terrible-tasting liquid form that comes from Herb Pharm.) If you know you have access to a local good health food store that carries bugleweed or lemon balm or motherwort, then you won't need to pick it up ahead of time.

I know that last paragraph sounds scary; it was designed to. You don't want to wander into something that you're not prepared for. Treating yourself comes with risks. But even if you can find someone to coach you through this, you need to know about what might happen as you try to figure yourself out.

Once a patient can take one pill or capsule of a thyroid supplement at breakfast and at lunch without negative results for two or three days, then the patient proceeds up to two in the morning and two at lunch, staying at that dose for a few days while monitoring symptoms. After two-and-two, the patient can try three-and-three, followed by four-and-four.

What if you do this and find that 70 percent of your symptoms go away with a dosage of three pills in the morning and three at noon? That's great, but now your job is to figure out how to get rid of your remaining symptoms. Most of us will be left with some issues that we can't figure out, but it's always best to shoot for 100 percent.

The next step might be to consider additional symptoms such as yeast overgrowth, adrenal fatigue, hormonal issues, a chronic infection, or anemia.

If you came into my clinic, I could personalize your treatment options to target exactly what you need. In this book I can only give you a condensed version of how I might help you in the clinic.

Iodine

This nutrient, critical for the production of thyroid hormone, is unlikely to need supplementation, since most people consume plenty of iodine in their diet from iodized salt or sea salt. Even though a number of thyroid health advocates recommend Lugol's solution or Iodoral (potassium iodide) as a source of iodine, I have not been overly impressed with using it in my clinical practice. My own experience shows that the better sources of supplementary iodine come from the iodine-rich seaweeds such as bladderwrack, kelp, or dulse.

L-tyrosine

As the basic building block for all thyroid hormones, a deficiency of the amino acid L-tyrosine will most definitely make it difficult for a person's thyroid to make adequate amounts of T4 and T3 hormone. However, because L-tyrosine should be present in most American diets, any shortage most likely stems from an inability to properly break down protein because of a stomach acid problem or a problem with absorption. To circumvent such a problem, you can buy L-tyrosine supplements, labeled by that name and available from most reputable supplement manufacturers.

Glandulars

"Glandular" supplements are derived from the gland tissue of animals, particularly cows (bovine glandulars) and pigs (porcine glandulars). Glandular supplements come from healthy glands, and the healthy glandular extract contains everything required for healthy gland function. When someone with an unhealthy gland supplements with the healthy glandular extract, the function of their own gland improves. Thyroid glandular supplements, which are free of all thyroid hormones, can be a very effective treatment for a hypothyroid condition.

Some people become squeamish at the idea of taking glandular preparations, especially when we start talking about neonatal glandulars (newborn animal glands). I understand, but I so much prefer natural over synthetic. God made that animal, and (fortunately for us) He used the same general design for them as He did for us. Try to get over it. The alternative to the glandular would have to be something from a chemistry lab.

Adrenal glandular (neonatal bovine)

Adrenal support supplements abound. DHEA is very commonly used by health care practitioners. Many herbalists prefer the ginsengs (Panex and Siberian) and licorice root. I like Biotics Research's Cytozyme AD better; I have not found anything else like it. If you are reading this and saying to yourself, "Well, I know adrenal glandulars aren't what I need because I've used them in the past and they didn't help," please find this one and try it.

Remember my analogy of the adrenal glands being like a bucket? I am always trying to figure out what is drilling holes in the bottom of someone's "adrenal bucket." Is it a food allergy or sensitivity? How about a viral infection? What is draining this person's emergency fund? After we figure it out, we deal with those issues. On top of that, I recommend Cytozyme AD, because it makes it all so much more humane.

What do I mean by that? Let me explain. One of the symptoms of low adrenal function is the tendency to make mountains out of molehills. Everything seems overwhelming. Life seems too hard. In adrenal fatigue, a person's emotions run his or her logic centers. So if a person starts filling his or her adrenal bucket immediately with Cytozyme AD, even though the bucket still has holes in it, all this extra work of changing diet or fighting a chronic viral infection seems a lot more achievable. In other words, with a more emotionally sound patient, you achieve better results.

Thyroid glandular (bovine or porcine)

(This should not be mistaken for Armour thyroid preparation, which has thyroid hormones in it.) When I want a product that is thyroid glandular only, I prefer the MBi Nutraceuticals bovine source, although the porcine glandular is OK too. I also choose Biotics Research GTA and GTA Forte (both porcine). For more complete information, see my Recommended Thyroid Supplements in Appendix C, "Dr. B's Suggestions."

Pituitary/hypothalamus glandular

In earlier chapters we spoke of how the hypothalamus and pituitary help control and regulate thyroid function. If I suspect that the reason for someone's thyroid dysfunction can be traced back to the pituitary or hypothalamus "prompter," then I recommend this glandular.

How would you know if yours is a hypothalamus or pituitary issue? Typically, since the pituitary gland also is responsible for stimulating the adrenal glands to secrete growth hormone, FSH (follicle-stimulating hormone), and LH (luteinizing hormones, which control egg release and development in women), a health evaluation can detect an increased need for these hormones in addition to thyroid hormones.

Also, one of the symptoms of a challenged pituitary gland is what I call the pituitary headache. The angled bony region of your face where your nose ends and becomes your forehead is called the glabella. The pituitary gland is situated straight back from the glabella, and it lies in a saddle-shaped bone about halfway back into your skull. Since most glands swell when they are over-challenged to do their work (remember our discussion of swollen thyroids—goiters—in chapter 5), so can the pituitary gland. Unfortunately, when a pituitary swells, it has nowhere to swell since it is trapped in a bony area. So the result is headache pain. In women, this type of headache will show up more often at certain times of their menstrual cycle.

To help with over-challenged pituitary and hypothalamus glands, I utilize Biotics Research's Cytozyme PT-HPT as a glandular supplement that has both bovine pituitary and hypothalamus extracts in it.

Supplements Specifically for Hypothyroidism

The following minerals can be effectively supplemented for hypothyroid patients:

Zinc

This mineral helps in thyroid production and T4 conversion to the more bioactive T3, but it also plays a role in improving communication between the thyroid hormones and the receptor sites of the cells they need to communicate with. It is also active in helping TRH (secreted from the hypothalamus gland) in communicating with the pituitary gland. It's best to find a zinc source that uses zinc bound with citrate, gluconate, glycinate, or (amino acid) chelate.

Selenium

This mineral helps the thyroid in producing T4 in the thyroid as well as assisting in the conversion of T4 to T3 once the hormones leave the thyroid. The other function of selenium is to improve the elimination of mercury from the system. As I detailed in chapter 7, mercury is known to inhibit proper thyroid function. Selenium helps because it competes antagonistically with mercury for absorption sites as well as helping the body excrete mercury. Selenium is also known to help with heart function and is an antioxidant (a substance that fights against free radical damage).

Copper

This mineral is critical in the production of T4 in the thyroid gland. It is also an essential mineral in the making of red blood cells. So it's always possible that having a copper deficiency could cause some type of anemia. There are almost too many sources of copper in our daily lives, and because copper and zinc compete with each other in your body, an excess of copper can cause a deficiency of zinc. Watch how much copper you're getting in relation to the zinc.

Calcium and magnesium

Neither of these nutrients contributes directly to thyroid function, but inadequate levels can create problems. For example, if you have been hypothyroid for a long time and your body has never seen a normal level of T4 and/or T3, your heart might be prone to beat irregularly if your magnesium and/or calcium levels are low. Read on to find out why they may be low and what to do about it.

Escaping the Vicious Circle

Since copper, selenium, zinc, and rubidium are all required for proper thyroid function, we often find a vicious circle with regard to stomach acid. Low thyroid function contributes to low hydrochloric acid production, which inhibits absorption of vital minerals, which further contributes to the body's hypothyroidism. Round and round we go. Also, since the amino acid L-tyrosine is the core building block of thyroid hormone, and amino acids are made from protein and protein requires hydrochloric acid to be broken down in the stomach, we certainly have another reason to restore the body's hydrochloric acid production and secretion.

The solution to this problem is to support and heal the person's system until the thyroid can work (if it can) on its own. Foods that turn out to be injuring the stomach lining (i.e., food allergies and sensitivities) need to be eliminated from the person's diet. No sense creating more repair work than is necessary for the poor thyroid. The person may need to supplement his or her output of hydrochloric acid temporarily. I am not a believer in long-term hydrochloric acid supplementation, but sometimes people need to help their bodies catch up.

Calcium, magnesium, and potassium are key nutrients in muscle contraction and relaxation. For instance, did you know that if you have chronic muscle-cramping or any localized muscle-twitching, you almost assuredly have a deficiency of calcium, magnesium, or potassium (or some combination of two or all three)? In some instances, the body is deficient in calcium, magnesium, or potassium, and that causes the heart to overreact.

One the big challenges with treating hypothyroid patients is getting enough hormone into their systems without causing their hearts to freak out. I find that if I am stimulating the thyroid enough, but there's not enough conversion to T3 taking place, the heart will start beating too fast or feel like it's beating "out of the patient's chest." This indicates that I need to work on helping the conversion to T3 to take place.

Certainly there are other nutrients that have a health benefit on the heart: CoQ_{10} (coenzyme Q_{10}), taurine, the components of Heart Terrain (from Apex Energetics), and omega-3 fatty acids (from fish or fish oil or flaxseed oil).

These heart-helpful nutrients are often inadequate in hypothyroid patients because too often the stomach (like the rest of their body) is not being routinely repaired or healed very well. In the healthy stomach, the cells of the lining of the stomach make and release hydrochloric acid and pepsinogen, which help with the absorption of nutrients from the gastrointestinal tract. If your body's production of hydrochloric acid is low, your absorption of nutrients will be low, which will complicate your ability to benefit from supplementation.

In addition, if a hypoactive pituitary is contributing to the hypothyroidism, this would be another reason for low hydrochloric acid. The release of the hormone gastrin (the major hormone that regulates acid secretion in the stomach) is stimulated by the pituitary gland. So if we see low hydrochloric acid, low growth hormone, low adrenals, (all hormones released by the pituitary), or irregular/

dysfunctional menstrual cycles, we may suspect that we need to support the pituitary gland.

All of the minerals that your body needs require hydrochloric acid in order to be absorbed. If a person's body isn't making enough hydrochloric acid, I find that quite often food allergies or sensitivities have been irritating the stomach lining to the point of damaging the parietal cells that make hydrochloric acid. By eliminating the irritating foods, stomach acid production increases and mineral absorption increases, thereby reducing the need for mineral supplementation.

If a wide variety of minerals are deficient and you suspect that low stomach acid is impeding mineral absorption, you may need supplementation with hydrochloric acid in the form of betaine HCl supplements. Symptoms of low stomach acid include belching or gas within an hour of eating, bloating shortly after eating, and even feeling full far longer than you think you should after a meal.

In my office I supply patients with a "hydrochloric acid challenge test" to see if they can benefit from this. Patients who have a lot of mineral deficiencies find that a hydrochloric acid deficiency needs to be a core treatment protocol. Otherwise they end up taking three or four times more of each mineral (iron, calcium, magnesium, selenium, manganese, rubidium, zinc, etc.) in order to be able to absorb normal amounts. It only makes sense to deal with their impaired digestion/absorption instead of taking massive amounts of minerals.

Solutions for Related Problems

Since the human body is so complex and all of its systems are so interrelated, any treatment of thyroid dysfunction must address the cause-and-effect nature of other health problems. In my clinical practice, I find that thyroid patients often present one or more of the following symptoms to which I need to offer solutions.

Depression

Many cases of depression are helped by fixing an underactive thyroid or cases of adrenal fatigue. L-tyrosine has been used for years as a natural remedy to assist in the treatment of depression, and L-tyrosine happens to be second in importance to only iodine in the creation of thyroid hormone. Of course there are several nutrients and herbs that are very effective for treating depression. Some rival the effectiveness of pharmaceutical drugs and have been shown in studies to be equally effective, but without all the side effects. I will use them to help patients.

However, as you know by now, my preference is to figure out if there is an underlying physical issue that is causing the depression. That problem could be physical or emotional, so I prefer fixing that underlying issue or issues first before we decide how to manage the depression. Hypothyroid patients definitely have a higher rate of depression than the normal population. If we address the thyroid, the energy goes up and the brain function improves.

It is my contention that a strong majority of cases of postpartum depression are simply the result of a low-functioning thyroid, adrenal fatigue, or just plain nutrient depletion. Let's face it; during pregnancy the baby takes everything and the mom gets what's left. And if the mother's body has been subjected to early trimester morning sickness, it's very difficult for her to catch up nutritionally during the final four to six months of pregnancy.

To not only help with pregnancy but also to head off postpartum deficiencies, I recommend Clinical Nutrients Prenatal during pregnancy. I find it to be far better than most ob-gyn-recommended nutritional supplements. You should be able to find it at a full service pharmacy or a health food store. (The company used to be Phyto Pharmica, but now it is sold under the Integrative Therapeutics brand name.)

Gallbladder dysfunction

A sluggish or congested gallbladder is sometimes called biliary (meaning having to do with bile) stasis (not moving). I listed the symptoms in chapter 5. Biotics Research Beta TCP is my supplement of choice, and its main ingredient is beet extract. Some people might say, "I like beets. Can I just eat beets?" The answer is, "Not likely." The beet extract is concentrated, and beets themselves contain a lot of sugar. By the time you would eat enough beets to equal my dosage of Beta TCP, you'd be sick or massively overweight. Beta TCP has beet, L-taurine, and pancrelipase in it. It helps the gallbladder bile get moving again. The challenging part of using Beta TCP is that it helps to high-dose this at four to seven tablets three times per day, which seems like a lot.

A little over half the time, I also include liquid iodine (aqueous potassium iodide) in the gallbladder regimen, because it serves as a thinner that works for a congested gallbladder as well as for sinus/inner ear congestion.

Yeast overgrowth

Do you remember the weed and seed analogy from chapter 5? To eliminate the "weeds," choose a nutritional/herbal product formulated as an antifungal. I use Candicid Forte (by Ortho Molecular) and FC-Cidal (by Biotics Research) as well as a fungal-yeast preparation that is supplied by DC Nutrition. As for "seed," you just need to find some good probiotics and not be afraid to take too many of them. If you have a great many symptoms of yeast and believe you have had them for some time, you may have one of the predisposing factors that perpetuate the growth of yeast in the human body: excess estrogen, low body pH (check your saliva and urine using litmus paper; a normal pH should be between 6.5 and 7.0), and low body oxygen (seen easily with pulse oximetry).

Female dysfunction/infertility

I use different combinations of products here, including dong quai (especially as it is supplied via Equi-Fem by Biotics Research) and progesterone. The progesterone can be in the sublingual form or cream. I wish I could provide you with a comprehensive list of good creams and liquids, but the list would quickly become obsolete. My best suggestion would be to go to our clinic's website or to do a Google search for an up-to-date list of quality progesterone products Two great books on progesterone treatment are *What Your Doctor May Not Tell You About Menopause* and *Hormone Balance Made Simple*, both by the late Dr. John R. Lee.

Vitamin A deficiency

Most people do not have a vitamin A deficiency as a primary problem. But if the thyroid has been underfunctioning for a while and consequently beta-carotene has not been getting converted by the thyroid into vitamin A, we may need to jump-start the thyroid gland. Or if the person's gallbladder has been sluggish and not properly processing fats, fat-soluble vitamins might not be absorbed properly, thereby causing the person to become deficient in vitamin A, vitamin D, vitamin K, and d-alpha tocopherol. Some omega-3 fatty acids could be deficient also from poor assimilation. Cases of longstanding chronic viral infections could also explain the deficiency because of vitamin A's effect with regard to supporting the immune system during viral infections. A vitamin A deficiency is easy to treat, but a patient can reach a toxic level if they aren't careful to monitor themselves. Some symptoms of excess vitamin A include headaches or itchy skin. Lab tests may even show the liver to show signs of reversible inflammation.

Anemia

Anemia is a deficiency of iron. I strongly recommend that, because an individual can become overloaded on iron without even knowing it, you have your family doctor run an iron panel blood test before you take additional iron. An iron panel tests for serum iron, ferritin, CBC (complete blood count), transferrin, and TIBC (total iron-binding capacity).

Once you find out your iron levels are low and you have hypothyroidism, you have a few options. You can increase your intake of iron (for example, from red meat, liver, eggs, spinach, kale, raisins, molasses, and grape juice/wine). There is also evidence that cooking in a cast iron skillet will increase the iron content of your food.

The next option is to supplement with iron. The best sources of iron are iron citrate, iron gluconate, iron fumarate, and iron succinate. You will find that supplements for these forms of iron will supply about 20–25 mg of iron. If your iron deficit is very large, you may require a prescription form such as ferrous sulfate (300+ mg per tablet), although this iron supplement tends to be very hard on the gastrointestinal tract. You will need to discontinue if you experience bad stomach pains or constipation.

Your stools will almost always turn black when you are taking an iron supplement. Don't worry about that. My only concern with black stools is that you can't tell the difference between iron-supplement black stools and black stools that stem from a bad upper gastrointestinal bleed. Also common with iron supplementation is constipation. If you become constipated, you can take a laxative on a short-term basis, while you're taking the iron supplement, but try not to take it long term.

You should never take iron if your transferrin levels are low, because that means your bloodstream will have no way to carry the iron around in your body. You also don't want to take iron if you're anemic but your ferritin levels are normal or high. It means you already have plenty of iron, but you probably can't make good red blood cells for a different reason.

Note that you should always take iron with meals to avoid stomach issues. And request an iron panel to make sure that your body is assimilating the iron and that your ferritin is increasing, along with your iron, hemoglobin, hematocrit, and red blood cell levels. Some iron is good, but excess iron is bad. Elevated ferritin levels have been shown to be a risk factor (like blood pressure and total cholesterol) for heart disease. This is why follow-up blood work is always important.

Since you usually do not know exactly why your system became depleted and anemic, I usually recommend that patients without access to an office visit take anemia supplements. Examples include Hemagenics from Metagenics and Fe-zyme from Biotics Research. Make sure that the supplement you choose contains at least vitamin C, copper, vitamin B_{12}, and folic acid in addition to an absorbable form of iron.[3]

A few other supplements might be helpful. If you've had blood work done and your globulin is low (< 3.0) then I would recommend taking some spleen glandular. If your body needs hydrochloric acid or you're anemic and the blood test (CBC) shows the average size of the red cell to be larger than normal (MCV >95), you may find it necessary to supplement with vitamin B_{12} instead of iron. Copper and/or folic acid can be helpful if the vitamin B_{12} doesn't help.

Chronic viral infection

Unfortunately, this topic is a book unto itself. Some viral infections last a lifetime. Herpes never goes away. (There is an oral version of this as well as a genital version.) Chicken pox is a childhood infection, but in many people the varicella virus goes into hiding, and then, later on in life when the immune system no longer considers it a threat, the virus produces symptoms again. This condition is called herpes zoster; most people know it as shingles. Other chronic viruses include Epstein-Barr, which causes infectious mononucleosis but many times continues "bugging" the system for years. Cytomegalovirus is another virus in this same group and can wreak havoc when the immune system is running low.

Some good treatment options include ascorbic acid, zinc, and L-lysine; all three are great for any herpes infection. Lauric acid, extracted from coconut oil, is also present in human breast milk. It is believed to strip the outside cell layer from viruses hiding from the immune system so that the body can mount an effective immune response. Thymus glandular and spleen glandular are good at improving the immune system. Echinacea is always a good standby. Lomatium and astragalus are other herbs known to improve the body's viral defenses.

Good formulations include Ortho Molecular's Viracid, Ecological Formula's Monolaurin, Med-Chem Lab's Lauricidin, Bio-Immunozyme Forte from Biotics Research, and Herb Pharm's Virattack.

Taking Care of Your Body

Your body is wonderfully complex. Everything is interrelated. God made it that way. In a perfect world, we would not need to work so hard to remedy the deficiencies and weaknesses that accumulate over time, because our bodies would not be subject to the extreme stresses (self-imposed and from the outside) that weaken our body's systems.

Since we live in a very imperfect world, we must grapple with problem after problem in the realm of health. But we can help each other conquer our many health problems, and that is what I have been trying to do for you in this book. Please be sure so spend some time exploring "Dr. B's Suggestions" in Appendix C. That is where I have collected many of the helpful details referred to in this chapter and others.

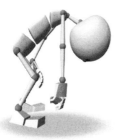

Chapter 10

STRUGGLES WITH WEIGHT

This book is really not meant to be a weight-loss book, but I know that many of you who suffer with hypothyroidism have issues with weight.

If you want to lose weight but you're not ready to make a lifetime change, then stop right now. If you want to lose weight so you can fit into your old drum and bugle corps marching band uniform for your fifteenth reunion, then skip it. I don't really want to help you do that. I know it sounds weird to say that, but many recent studies have shown that yo-yo dieting is harder on the human body than just staying fat. Plus, I have quite a problem with people who spend months or years losing eighty pounds only to gain back all of it, or more, in half the time it took them to lose it. It breaks my heart. So if you aren't ready to make the commitment to lose weight and keep it off, please don't start.

But if you're serious about eating right to get healthy and you have thyroid issues, you need to first start eating more protein. With all the material that I've presented in this book, one thing should become very apparent to you: I believe that we in America eat too many carbohydrates. We eat too much food…period, but we definitely eat too many carbohydrates. The whole point of eating carbohydrates (sugars or starches) is to provide fuel for the system to function on. Since most of us in the United States don't do much physical work compared to the rest of the world, we don't need fuel.

Storing More Than We Need

Let me present a hypothetical situation to you. I am struggling with garage space. I no longer have any room for a car. I have a 2.5 car garage but I am thinking of buying the adjacent lot next to me so I can expand my garage, and then I'll have room for my car. What? You have questions for me? OK. What am I storing in my garage? Same things as everyone else. I have a hand-push lawn mower, a snow shovel, a rake, and 139 five-gallon gas containers, all entirely full. What do you mean when you ask me, "Why do you have so many containers for gas?" Where else would I put all my extra gas? Each one of those containers is full. Huh?

OK. I can see you're confused, although I'm not sure why. Let me explain. My car needs gas. My tank takes fifteen gallons of fuel. Each time I go out and use my car, I buy fifteen gallons of gas because that's what the manufacturer tells me is my fuel tank capacity. Where am I driving in my car? I'm really lucky. I have a grocery store only four blocks from my house, and it has a gas station right next to it. A lot of times my tank is too full for all the extra gas, so I just buy a couple of five-gallon containers... you know, those nice red ones with the gas spout hidden inside it. Anyway, I fill up a few of those, and I store them inside my garage. In case you can't tell from your vantage point, I have five-gallon jugs floor to ceiling about three layers thick lining my garage. So, can you see the reason that I need to build an addition to my current garage?

OK. If this was a real conversation, you'd think I was an idiot, right? Why on earth would I buy that much gas and store it? But we do the same thing with regard to carbohydrates. We need just a tiny amount of fuel to sit in front of the television or surf on the computer. Even if you are a mom of little kids and you really do work hard (I'm serious, I know you do), you're still not burning that much fuel changing diapers, wiping noses, picking up kids and putting them in their high chairs, etc. It's hard work, but it's not burning that much fuel. Let's be clear: our ancestors did hard physical work, but we don't.

So have I made myself clear? Our current society does the least amount of physical, fuel-burning work than any other time in the history of known civilization, and we eat more than at any time in the history of the world. Do you see the reason for the "layers of gas" lining the inside of our "garages"? We sit on the brink of disaster. We have an epidemic level of obesity. You might be concerned about my garage and what an incendiary, explosive situation it could be, but we should be equally concerned about the level of obesity in America. It is easily the number one problem at the core of a variety of diseases. And we refuse to acknowledge it. The average male consumes about 2,475 calories per day, while the average female consumes 1,833 calories. It has been estimated that since 1970, we eat 525 more calories than we did back then (and to reiterate, we are burning less).

What is a calorie? You hear the word all the time. When we say calorie, we are actually referring to a kilocalorie, or 1,000 calories. The calorie is the amount of energy required to raise one gram of water one degree centigrade. It's potential energy. All the dieticians have clamored over fat as the evil because each gram of fat has 9 calories when each gram of carbohydrate or gram of protein has only 4 calories. So for a plateful of food, you will get less calories (potential energy) from it if the fat content of the food is lower. More bang for your buck, so to speak.

Carbs: The Pros and Cons

The nice part about carbohydrates is that they burn clean. We hear of natural gas as clean burning compared to coal. Here is what they are saying: once the potential energy has been gleaned from each, the natural gas has released carbon dioxide and water into the environment, while the coal released carbon dioxide and sulfur products. Carbohydrates are similar to natural gas. When we burn them, we are left with carbon dioxide and water. Very clean. If we burn protein as fuel or fat as fuel, we have more waste materials that we have to account for and get rid of.

The bad part about carbohydrates is that they are nature's way of providing us with quick fuel. The fancy term for this is that they have a *high glycemic index.* This means they form sugar fairly quickly. Sugar and high-fructose corn syrup are very close to usable sugar and thereby have high glycemic indexes. Starches are nature's storage form for usable sugar. Starch is basically a long chain of glucose molecules. Glucose molecules are the fuel of the human body. Every time we need fuel, the body tries to convert the fat, protein, starch, and fruit sugar called fructose into glucose. In case you're keeping track, I haven't gotten to the bad part yet. Here it is, though. If the body provides us sugar, it's expecting us to need to burn the sugar. The other possibility the body will consider is that you are in a time of plentiful food. It's harvest time, and you are packing food away so that you will have something to live on during the lean winter/spring months. Feast now, famine later. In America, we are always in the feast mode, storing for a famine that will never happen.

How does the body do this? It sees that the sugar is rising too high, and it assumes that you are feasting for "later." Elevated glucose levels trigger the beta cells of Langerhans of the pancreas to secrete insulin. Insulin's job is simply to get the sugar out of the bloodstream. It does so in three ways. First, it tries to find a cell that wants it/needs it. The best way to remember what insulin does is to just picture it as being the sugar/fat key. It unlocks the doors to the cells of the body to allow sugar to go in. So the first most likely place is any cell that needs sugar. If there aren't any, it goes to Plan B. Insulin stimulates the liver cells to turn some of the excess glucose into a starch called glycogen. There aren't many storage places for glycogen in the body (muscles and liver), but glycogen can provide a quick source of fuel in between meals if the body starts running low. If, after the body has made glycogen, there's still an elevated sugar level, the body sends the remaining sugar into the liver to be turned into triglycerides. You may remember that word from a blood test or someone talking about cholesterol and they happen to mention triglycerides. The triglycerides are released back into the bloodstream, and the insulin then acts as a key to help the triglycerides get into the fat cells so we'll have some energy source once the famine hits.

Here's the odd thing. You've probably heard of the Atkin's Diet or Protein Power, or the South Beach Diet…the list goes on and on of low-carbohydrate diets. The reason these diets work is that we trick the system. Protein will stimulate the body to make a small amount of insulin, but not anywhere near what it does when elevated glucose is around. So if we can keep the carbohydrate level low, or keep the glycemic index low, the insulin won't get secreted and the body won't go into storage mode.

Here's another really strange fact. Did you know that if I ate nothing but butter, lard, olive oil, whipping cream…if my diet was 100 percent fat without any protein or carbohydrates, my body would starve and I'd die just as if I wasn't eating anything. It's documented in almost every biochemistry textbook. The reason is, my body's insulin will not let any sugar in any cells because of the absence of insulin. Despite consuming a food that has twice the potential energy by weight, I wouldn't be able to utilize it.

I know. You thought this was a chapter on weight loss. I needed to be able to have you get your head around the concept that for most of us, "carbohydrates are bad." The exceptions out there are any of you who are at a good weight and with a cholesterol level that is less than 170 and a triglyceride level less than 80. You guys burn through and rarely have any excess glucose to store. The rest of us need to eat less overall and have a higher percentage as protein/veggies if we are to lose weight and keep it off.

That leads me to my next explanation: whatever you do to lose weight, you need to be able to keep it up long term. If you can't, don't use that weight-loss program. It will eventually fail. If all you can think about while you're on the program is how great it will be to be off the program and eating "normally" again, don't do it.

It's Not a Sprint;
It's a Marathon

There are a number of good programs out there. My guess is that to do what I've been teaching you in this book, you'll need to modify some of the "good foods" in each of the programs to be your "good foods." Artificial sweeteners are not good foods. White flour is not good food. Sugar and high-fructose corn syrup are not good foods.

What I am going to tell you is the same thing that I've been telling you since the first chapter of this book. You need to listen to your body. It will show you by losing weight and by your energy and well-being how your diet is going and how much food is the right amount. Weight Watchers is a good program if you are interested in having an accountability group and to find out how many calories you should be eating (and you want the calculation to be easy). It is a point-based system that gives foods points and gives you a number of points per day that you are allowed; it also gives you extra points each week that you have in order to have a binge day or to add to each of your daily points. I did four months of Weight Watchers at one point with my wife because every patient who came to me and told me they did Weight Watchers lost weight on it. What I found helpful on the program was knowing how much food was OK for a guy my age, my size, and with my level of activity. My caloric maintenance level is about 2,100 calories per day and thirty Weight Watcher points a day. There is a website that can give you a variety of information, including how many calories you should be eating per day (www.freedieting.com). It also gives a basic idea as to a wide spectrum of diets with the pros or cons of each. There is also a wide assortment of apps for Android and iPhone compatible devices that can give you diets and maybe even a menu/shopping list for the week. Again, the challenge might be using their meal plan. They may say it's fine having a slice of white bread where I'm saying that it's not. I have read the book *The Paleo Solution* and listened to the author's podcasts, and although I don't necessarily buy into the "when we were cavemen" explanation, I believe the diet would most closely resemble what I am sharing with you in this book.

Again, I know that this is not a weight-loss book. I'm not trying to make it weight-loss book. However, I would be remiss if I didn't acknowledge that, if you are overweight, it is one of the top issues that you would like to see resolved. I know you've also probably done diets and exercise plans, only to have them fail. You need to try again. The difference is that this time you will be supporting your system and listening to your system.

The Heart of the Matter

In the King James Version of the Bible, Paul talks about buffeting his body. Some jokes have been made by preachers/leaders who turn the word *buffet* into an all-you-can-eat smorgasbord to imply that Paul was saying one of his spiritual disciplines was overeating. And you know what? I get the joke. And, if it wasn't so true and sadly epidemic, I might find it more amusing. I like a good pun as much as the next guy. My wife and kids might even roll their eyes at this and say "significantly more than the next guy." However, gluttony is not a laughing matter; it's a sin. It's referred to several times in the Bible. Sometimes it's even paired with drunkenness.

The Bible doesn't say that money is the root of evil; it says the *love* of money, the heart issue behind the money, is the root of evil. By the same token, eating is not sinful; it's the heart issue behind it. Gluttony is not simply eating a lot of food. Gluttony is the "eating for all the wrong reasons." Feeding cravings. Emotional eating. It implies that what my body wants, it gets. It masters me. I don't master it.

I know someone whose pastor always used to say, "There's no meetin' without eatin'." However, I think we need to remember that no matter what you eat or drink, do so to the glory of God. (See 1 Corinthians 10:31.) Jesus relaxed and ate with people. Food is a great way to gather together. It's been suggested that even Communion was simply that, gathering for a meal to remember Jesus and be a community and share and be connected with each other.

In Closing

It may seem that I've been all over the map in this chapter, but I'm trying to fit what I believe could fill an entire book into a chapter. In summary, here's what I believe you need to know to lose weight:

1. Remember first and foremost that you are beautiful and/or handsome whether or not you lose weight. You should not be losing weight to become more desirable or lovable.

2. We are responsible for doing what we believe God is showing us to do. God is responsible for the results.

3. Drink plenty of good, pure water.

4. Get some cardiovascular exercise (something that increases your heart rate) for thirty to sixty minutes at least three times a week, and add some resistance training (weights) into it if possible.

5. Go predominantly with eating protein and veggies with some fruits (avoid or limit starchy veggies like potatoes and corn).

6. Find your calorie limit necessary to lose weight, and learn to be satisfied with that amount of food.

7. Take something to boost your thyroid function if, based on this book, you believe you have a low-functioning thyroid.

8. Do not be afraid, anxious, or concerned about anything. Do what you know you're supposed to do, and remember that God is in control.

9. Food is good. God made food delicious and wholesome. We just need to eat God's food and not man's adulterated, genetically modified version of food. And for the last time, *food is not made in a chemistry lab!*

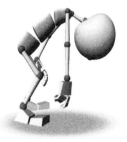

Chapter 11

THE BODY IS ALWAYS RIGHT

I f I had a recipe for birthday cake that came out right only once every five or six times I made it, I would try to find new recipe.

That's why I decided to try to find a new master "recipe" for my patients whose thyroid function came out too low or too high (or somewhere in between, with fluctuating symptoms of dysfunction). When I started out, all of the medical professionals in my area seemed to think that the thyroid-stimulating hormone (TSH) test was a great evaluator of thyroid function. But I had to wonder...if it was such a great diagnostic tool, why did it fail to deliver useful information more than half of the time? Surely this pointed to a need for a better approach to a widespread problem. Too many people needed help, right now. I couldn't ignore them.

I decided to disagree with the experts. Some might think that sounds cocky, but I call it stupid to keep following formulas that only work every now and then.

I am not a research-based practitioner. Of course, I read up on what people are trying and what they say as valid. But most of the time I put it through my "God filter" before I decide what to do. If it makes sense to me and I have a peace about it, and if it points back to God's original plan for the human body, then I will try it out on some patients.

As I have been saying throughout the preceding chapters of this book, I generally do not believe in tricking the body with work-arounds, jerry-rigging natural bodily functions, or providing for the body what it should be making on its own. I believe in supporting the body. My healing philosophy is to find out what is in the body that shouldn't be there (allergies/sensitivities, toxins, infections, excesses, and so forth) and come up with ways to remove it. At the same time I look for what seems to be missing in the body (the deficiencies) and try to find ways to supply what each unique human body needs for healthy performance.

If what I am doing doesn't work, I stop doing it. If it does work, I have no need to prove to scientists by means of burdensome studies that what I'm doing is working. I just need to remember what I did, learn from the results, and believe that it makes sense to try it again (if it proved successful). My philosophy of treatment and my techniques for applying it free me up. I can treat people as individuals who come with unique life situations. Sometimes I may need to create an unusual solution—and I'm free to do that.

People vary so much. Each individual comes with a different body type and different strengths and weaknesses. The challenge for me as a doctor is to spend enough time with each of my patients to "get" them. I need to assimilate what they have indicated on their history forms. I also need to observe, through interactions, each person's personality type. I cannot design an effective protocol for treatment unless I understand how my patient's attributes affect the way he or she tends to attack the challenges and issues of life.

Rebel With a Cause

I think it takes a certain personality type to rebel against the status quo with an attempt to make reforms. The German Christian reformer Martin Luther was like that. Hungarian doctor Ignaz Semmelweis probably had that kind of personality too. He's the one who insisted, while working in Vienna, that patients were dying because of the doctors' contaminated hands.[1] They were doing autopsies and then going on their rounds to examine the live patients without washing their hands.

Sometimes all it takes is a single well-placed action. Rosa Parks had likely gone to the back of the bus many times, but one day she decided not to go back there anymore. She was a rebel with a cause.

Now I am not trying to say that what I do is anywhere near the league of these people. Still, there are people suffering for lack of knowledge, and I know I am not alone in preaching this good news of hope and healing. Others are talking and writing about this approach to health, in particular this approach to thyroid issues. Broda Barnes developed his basal temperature diagnostic. Mary Shomon and Janie Bowthorpe, authors and patient advocates (in book and Web form), aim for a better approach to health care, encouraging people to expect good care from their doctors and to "fire" them if they don't receive it. Datis Kharrazian, health practitioner, author, and lecturer, is going around the country teaching the message of his book: *Why Do I Still Have Thyroid Symptoms When My Lab Tests Are Normal?* He talks about the failure of blood testing, and he is a research guru who can validate his message.

As for me, I have spent twenty years helping people to overcome their sickness in order to become the people God has called them to be. Although I say I do not like rules, I do like rules that are designed to protect me or protect others. Don't jump off the roof. Resist taking out your own appendix. These are very good rules. But I do not like hoops to jump through. I don't like rules that are not based in common sense.

I realize that some of you like rules because they make you feel safe. They reassure you that you are not wrong. But I prefer my common sense over rules. My wife gets irked with me because her common sense says not to wash the sharp knives by gliding her fingers down the flat sides of the knife—which is the *only* way I will wash a sharp knife. Naturally, she thinks that I'm going to hurt myself. Well, so far I have never cut myself in twenty years of doing dishes that way. Now, mind you, I did not choose this knife-washing method simply to express rebellion. I have a good reason, which is this: my bare fingertips can best feel whether or not I have cleaned all the debris off the knife. If I use a sponge or a cloth, I can't be as sure that the knife has gotten clean enough.

I have reasons why I do not follow other rules. Sometimes my reason is basic impatience. If I'm sitting at a stoplight in a quiet neighborhood at 1:00 a.m. for thirty seconds and there is no one in sight in any direction, I'm just going to go in spite of the red light. Yes, I know I break the law when I do that. But I figure that the stoplight is there to regulate traffic by allowing cars to take turns crossing that intersection. If I see no other cars to take turns with, why do I need to wait? Yes, I also know that if a cop happens to be sitting there waiting for a rule-breaker such as me, I will be fined for my traffic violation. But I'm willing to take that risk.

Taking People Seriously

Many times my patients tell me stories of prior visits to a doctor. They report what the doctor said when they explained their symptoms. In essence, "That can't happen."

A woman recounts: "It seems as though every time I talk on my cell phone, I get a headache. Is it possible that I have an issue with my cell phone?"

Doctor's response: "No. There have been many studies, and there is no correlation with brain issues and cell phone usage."

Really? This patient is trying to link things together, and the doctor shuts her down based on abstracts of studies? On this same premise, some doctors put their patients on antidepressants or anti-anxiety pills once they do a few tests and nothing shows up, essentially saying, "Since I know everything there is to know about the body, if I run some tests and can't find the problem, it must be that the patient is psychologically causing the problem." To me, that seems pretty arrogant.

Refusing to Play the Blame Game

True enough, patients can get it wrong. People like to play the victim card. "This awful, terrible thing has happened to me. How unfair. How terrible. None of it is my fault. I couldn't have done anything to stop this from happening to me." This conveniently deflects blame and judgment, and it also exempts the person from making any changes.

The medical system doesn't help when it blames your gene pool. "You have depression; you can't help it." "Your cholesterol is elevated, and you inherited the tendency.

True, none of that may be "fair." But I tell my patients: "This is the hand you've been dealt. Play it out to the best of your ability. You can whine about it—or you can try to make the best of it. I will help you, if you want me to."

In most cases, we have participated in our own demise. We were not born damaged. Well, OK, each of us carries a unique genetic code, and some people were born with physiological birth defects, visible and invisible. But *most* of us were not born with compromised health. Yet while we were still in the womb and very soon after our birth, our parents began to make decisions that affected our health. Soon we bought into those early decisions and the ones that came later. I do not need to tell you that many of the things that society promotes may be detrimental to our health down the road. We assume things are safe because people say so or because we want them to be safe, but in truth, all of them may hold some risk for some individuals.

Controversies abound. Even if it's after the fact for you, you need to come to informed conclusions about the relative risks of health procedures that are common in the United States. For example, consider the following:

Diagnostic ultrasounds during pregnancy

Ultrasound employs sound waves. We know that X-rays and other wave forms can affect the fragile genetic proteins of DNA. People who are concerned about the effects of ultrasound procedures during pregnancy quote a World Health Organization and US Department of Health and Human Services report: "It is not clear at this time whether ultrasound fetal monitoring is beneficial to the mother or fetus in terms of pregnancy outcome.... If there is no generally acknowledged benefit to the monitoring, there is no reason to expose patients to increased cost and risk. The question of benefit has not yet been resolved...and the potential for delayed effects has been virtually ignored."[2]

C-sections

I do not bring this up to make you worried about having a Caesarian birth if your child is in true fetal distress and needs to be born safely and quickly. However, C-sections are major surgery, and too many of them are scheduled for the sake of convenience and unnecessary fear. Childbirth is not a medical procedure; it is a miracle. Women should learn about C-sections both from those who promote the procedure and from those who are concerned about its popularity.

Vaccines

To vaccinate or not? This is another nice little polarizing, potentially life-changing decision that parents have to make. I have had patients whose children developed problems seemingly in close connection with a vaccination. Others, of course, have had no repercussions, only the beneficial protection from the disease against which the child was vaccinated. To weigh the decision, parents need to decide which is worse—the potential risks of a vaccination (which may cause autism) and the likelihood of the child catching the disease the vaccine has been designed to combat. The only good decision is an informed one.

Breast milk vs. infant formula

This is another decision that we make early on that can make a dramatic difference in the health of our children. As most people know, every study ever done that compares natural nursing to bottle-fed formula shows breastfeeding to be superior. The only glitch is that so many advice-givers remain convinced that some breastfeeding mothers need to supplement their insufficient supply of milk. Somehow the experts ignore the fact that a woman's own milk supply can be increased. (Isn't it crazy that we spend millions of dollars to help cows triple their milk supply on dairy farms, but we push women to significantly inferior infant formula as soon as their babies do not seem to be getting enough to eat?)

Also, some mothers complain that their babies seem to spit up a great deal after nursing or they become colicky. Ninety-nine times out of a hundred, the simple solution involves taking a look at the mom's diet. If she eats a food that the baby finds objectionable and the baby's body indicates that adverse reaction by spitting up, her ideal choice would be an elimination diet to see what food or foods the baby is getting through her breast milk that may be causing the problem. The truth is that the baby's spitting up is a signal that the mother needs to take a look at her diet—not a signal that she needs to switch her baby to formula feedings.

Whatever our actual decisions, we need to remember that fear is not a good motivation. We must remember that God will help us make decisions that have health implications. And He wants decisive soldiers, not vacillating victims; conquerors, not complainers. In case you haven't yet noticed this in the Old Testament, you need to know that God is not a big fan of grumblers and complainers. And as we see in the New Testament, He looks for people to whom He has given much and who overcome obstacles so that they can be trusted with more. (See Luke 12:48.)

In addition, He has given us each other. Why? So that we can help each other. In the case of health decisions, we can help each other interpret the signals our bodies are giving us. I see that as my primary job. I spend all of my time figuring out what people's bodies are trying to tell them. I know that the body is always right, but I also know that it's all too easy to misinterpret its messages.

My job is to determine why somebody's body is acting the way it is. Then I can help the person decide how best to overcome the problem. Human anatomy is simple in function but very complicated in design. Our bodies are smart. They compensate for lacks. They adapt. This can make it harder for us to figure out cause and effect.

Rarely do my patient's problems come from their own malingering (making up problems in order to receive attention, time off work, or disability payments). Only occasionally do I see psychological problems manifesting as physical problems. I know that our bodies can communicate information to us because I participate in the conversation. I can "talk to the body" and figure out what it's trying to say and how it needs help.

I hope that reading this book has helped you improve your own instincts for knowing what your body is telling you. I hope I have expanded your options for both self-diagnosis and self-help. I hope that you will continue to use the tools I have placed into your hands. Whether your problems turn out to have thyroid implications or not, I hope that you have learned enough to consider the possibility before you spend time, effort, and money on treatments that miss the mark.

My goal in this book has been to help *you* to become the expert on *yourself*, with the help of doctors, books, websites, and other resources, and most of all with the help of the Holy Spirit, who can help you tell the difference between truth and falsehood. Keep learning as much as you can, and then make up your own mind what to do. I endorse and applaud your efforts!

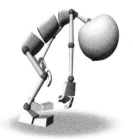

Appendix A

AXILLARY/BASAL TEMPERATURE TEST

1. Use an oral thermometer that has been shaken down to below 95°F and place on your bedside stand before going to sleep at night.[1]

2. On waking, place the thermometer in your arm pit for a full ten minutes. It is important to make as little movement as possible. Lying and resting with your eyes closed is best. Do not get up until the test is completed.

3. After ten minutes, read and record the temperature and date on the chart below.

4. Record the temperature for at least three mornings (preferably at the same time of day) and bring the information to your health care provider. (If there is a great fluctuation in temperatures, you may want to get more readings to get a more accurate assessment.) Women who are still having periods should perform the test on the second, third, and fourth days of their period. Men and postmenopausal women can perform the test at any time.

Date	Temperature

Date	Temperature

Add all of the temperatures together, and then divide them by the number of days you had a temperature reading. The normal range is 97.6 to 98.2. Hypothyroidism is any value less than 97.6 and is characterized by:

+ Chronic fatigue

+ Dry skin

+ Sensitive to cold

+ Cold hands/feet

+ Low sex drive

+ Constipation

+ Puffy/wrinkly skin

+ Slow reflexes

+ Excessive menstrual periods

+ Tendency toward PMS

+ Family history of goiters

+ Gaining weight easily

+ Chronically stiff joints

+ History of infertility

+ Trouble waking in the morning

+ Tendency toward depression/apathy

* Thinning or loss of outside of eyebrows

* Chronic anemia despite adequate iron intake

* Sugar-caused irritability and mood swings

* Chronically sore muscles

Medical treatment of hypothyroidism includes using a synthetic thyroid hormone replacement (T4) but does not provide for the other (more active) hormone T3. Consequently, patients on Synthroid may experience a mild improvement in fatigue and memory, but traditionally continue to be plagued with the remaining hypothyroid symptoms. The condition subclinical hypothyroidism is characterized by normal blood thyroid levels, along with over hypothyroid signs and symptoms.

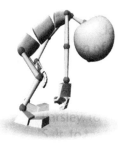

Appendix B

ARTIFICIAL SWEETENERS

To attain and maintain peak health, as you read in chapter 4 ("Healthy Eating"), you should avoid all artificial sweeteners. Here is an in-depth look at the most popular of the chemical sweeteners.

Saccharin

This product was discovered in a chemistry lab in the late nineteenth century by chemists who accidentally put their hands to their mouths and tasted the chemical they were working with. (I guess scientists were less concerned about the toxicity of their compounds in the 1870s than they are today.) It became more popular after there was a sugar shortage in World War I. It is sold primarily as Sweet'N Low, and people recognize it by its characteristic pink package in coffee shops and restaurants. It used to be the sweetener in diet soft drinks like Tab.

Because its aftertaste is much stronger than the newer sweeteners, its popularity has paled in comparison to the others. This is the only one of all the artificial sweeteners on the market that was forced to put a warning on the label stating that it caused cancer in laboratory rats. For this reason, one might think that this is therefore the worst of the artificial sweeteners, but it may be the least toxic of the three primary artificial sweeteners on the market.

NutraSweet (Aspartame)

This sweet chemical is two hundred times sweeter than sugar. Back in the 1990s, the labels of food companies would proudly state: "Made with NutraSweet." Its less-dominant aftertaste had soft drink manufacturers flocking to make a diet soda with it. Their marketing team made a big point of telling the world that their product was very "natural."

Of course it was composed of naturally occurring substances. But were they good for human bodies? NutraSweet is made by attaching two different amino acids, L-aspartic acid and L-phenylalanine.

This chemical sweetener was said to have been the most thoroughly tested food product ever in the history of the FDA. However, within a few years, NutraSweet held the record for most health complaints in the history of the FDA. In 1997, a book called *Excitoxins: The Taste that Kills*, written by Russell Blaylock, cited five hundred studies that had showed this "natural" sweetener to be much more toxic than previously believed. There is probably more than one reason for the toxicities, but a major problem with NutraSweet is that in certain patients it will break down into methanol. Does that name sound familiar?

Methanol is the alcohol present in what people call wood alcohol. You hear of people drinking methanol to get drunk (it can be present in higher amounts in homemade moonshine), but the breakdown product of methanol by alcohol dehydrogenase is formaldehyde, which further breaks down to formic acid. Formaldehyde and formic acid can produce nerve damage.

For this reason, NutraSweet has been called a neurotoxin for many people. Some have even been diagnosed with multiple sclerosis, only to discover later, after eliminating diet sodas, that most of their symptoms have disappeared.

Splenda (Sucralose)

Sucralose was discovered in 1975 by researchers at Queen Elizabeth College (now part of King's College London). It was discovered by Leslie Hough and a young Indian chemist Shashikant Phadnis. The duo were trying to make an insecticide. On a late-summer day, Phadnis was told to test the powder. Phadnis thought that Leslie asked him to taste it; so he did. He found the compound to be ridiculously sweet. The two worked with Tate & Lyle (a British sugar company) for a year before settling down on the final formula.[1]

Sucralose is a chlorinated sugar compound that is about six hundred times sweeter than sugar. In 1998 the FDA approved this chemical food to be introduced into our food supply. Initially, the Splenda public relations team put on the label, "Splenda is made from sugar, so it tastes like sugar." Yes, it's made from sugar, but it takes twenty-two steps chemically to replace those three oxygen atoms with chlorine atoms and to make them stay attached to the molecule that used to be sugar and not be broken down in the digestive tract.

Sucrose is the main sweetener in sugar. It is two sugars bound together: glucose and fructose. Its chemical structure is very basic. In comparison, here's Splenda (sucralose). I've seen the chemical name listed in two ways:

- 1,6-dideoxy-BETA-D-fructofuranosyl-4-chloro-4-deoxy-alpha-D-galactopyranoside

- 2-[2,5-bis(chloromethyl)-3,4-dihydroxyoxolan-2-yl]oxy-5-chloro-6-(hydroxymethyl)oxane-3,4-diol

Truthfully, this chemical we pour into our "diabetes-friendly" desserts and into "waist-conscious" coffee drinks is closer to the chemical structure of a pesticide than a food.

Research in animals has shown that sucralose can cause many problems, such as:

+ Shrunken thymus glands (up to 40 percent shrinkage)

+ Enlarged liver and kidneys

+ Atrophy of lymph follicles in the spleen and thymus

+ Increased cecal (a part of the colon) weight

+ Reduced growth rate

+ Decreased red blood cell count

+ Hyperplasia of the pelvis

+ Extension of the pregnancy period

+ Aborted pregnancy

+ Decreased fetal body weights and placental weights

+ Diarrhea

One of the selling points of Splenda was that it is not "absorbable," which was thought to limit the danger from any toxicity that may turn out to be verifiable. However, despite the manufacturer's claims to the contrary, sucralose seems to be absorbed to a significant degree, and it seems to be metabolized by the body. According to the FDA's "Final Rule" report, 11 to 27 percent of sucralose ingested is absorbed.[2] (The Japanese Food Sanitation Council estimates that as much as 40 percent of ingested sucralose gets absorbed.[3])

Most studies show that plasma sucralose has a half-life of from two to five hours, although its half-life in rabbits was found to be much longer, about thirty-six hours. After about 20 to 30 percent of the absorbed sucralose gets metabolized, both the metabolites and unchanged, absorbed sucralose are excreted in urine. The absorbed sucralose has been found to concentrate in the liver, kidney, and gastrointestinal tract. According to The Sucralose Toxicity Information Center, sucralose is broken down "into small amounts of 1,6-dichlorofructose, a chemical which has not been adequately tested in humans."[4]

Artificial sweeteners hide in food labels—even in organic products sometimes. As I found with hot chocolate mix (see chapter 4, "Healthy Eating"), even the version of a commercial product that is supposedly *not* the artificially sweetened one can have artificial sweeteners as an additional ingredient. If you want to avoid artificial sweeteners (or artificial anything), read food labels carefully.

Appendix C

DR. B'S SUGGESTIONS

This final section of the book is my effort to supply you with more information on some of the topics addressed in this book. Here, you will find the following:

+ Recommended Thyroid Supplements

+ The A-B-Cs of Calcium

+ Recommended Books About the Thyroid

+ Recommended Websites About the Thyroid

+ Where to Find Nutritionally Oriented Doctors

+ Selected Products That Contain Wheat and Sources for Alternatives to Wheat

+ "Eating Clean"—Selected Recipes and Tips

Recommended Thyroid Supplements

Once you have determined that there's enough evidence to suspect a low-functioning thyroid gland, you can begin to try supplementation. Most of the following supplements can be obtained from a variety online sources at competitive prices. (All of them can be found at www.notmedicine.com.) The following are the thyroid supplements that I use in my office.

Thyro Complex

I have used this product for years. It can help patients come off their prescription medications when their hormone levels are irregular. Although it contains a bit of kelp as a source of iodine, the primary active ingredients are the glandulars.

Ingredients:

- Iodine (from kelp), 900 mcg (600 percent DV)

- Raw bovine thyroid concentrate (thyroxin-free), 60 mg

- Raw adrenal concentrate (porcine), 30 mg

- Raw pituitary concentrate (porcine), 10 mg

- Raw spleen concentrate (porcine), 10 mg

- Kelp, 180 mg

Spectra 303T

This product seems to have the right blend of minerals, glandulars, and iodine. It's a bit pricey, but definitely worth it as a reliable help for hypothyroidism.

Ingredients:

- Iodine (kelp source [Ascophyllum nodosum]), 225 mcg (150 percent DV)

- Zinc (as zinc gluconate), 10 mg (67 percent DV)

- Copper (as copper gluconate), 500 mcg (25 percent DV)

- L-tyrosine, 100 mg (DV not established)

- Thyroid tissue (bovine source, thyroxine free), 100 mg (DV not established)

THY-O

This is a homeopathic preparation that is good at jump-starting thyroid glands that have been sluggish for a while.

Ingredients:

+ Thyroid 5C Native Gold 8X

+ Bloodtwig Dogberry (buds) 1DH

+ Sweet Almond (buds) 1DH

+ Black Currant (buds) 1DH

Thyroid-120

This supplement from MBi Nutraceuticals is very effective when I know that the thyroid gland needs glandular support only. This glandular is similar to the Armour prescription except that it contains bovine thyroid, not porcine, and Thyroid-120 does not have any hormone in it.

Ingredients:

+ Vitamin E, 2 IU

+ Pyridoxine HCl, 2 mg

+ New Zealand freeze-dried bovine thyroid tissue, 120 mg

Thyroid Plus drops

This is another homeopathic preparation, more subtle in its effects than THY-O, but great when the thyroid doesn't need a lot of stimulation.

Ingredients:

+ Fucus vesiculosus 4X

+ Natrum muriaticum 6X

+ Lycopus virginicus 6X

- Spongia tosta 4X

- Kalium iodatum 6X

- Calcarea iodata 6X

- Thyroid 6/1⅔0/60/200X

- Adrenal 6/1⅔0/60/200X

- Pituitary 6/1⅔0/60/200X

- Thymus 6/1⅔0/60/200X

- Spleen 6/1⅔0/60/200X

T-100

This is my strong thyroid booster. I use T-100 when I have a patient who has a long way to go and whose thyroid needs a great deal of stimulation. T-100 is the most likely to make the thyroid overshoot into hyperthyroidism.

Ingredients:

- Thyroid glandular (thyroxine free), 100 mg (DV not established)

- Adrenal glandular, 50 mg (DV not established)

- Pituitary glandular, 15 mg (DV not established)

- Spleen glandular, 5 mg (DV not established)

- Thymus glandular, 5 mg (DV not established)

- L-Tyrosine, 30 mg (DV not established)

- Dulse (Rhodymenia palmetta), 400 mg (DV not established)

- Bladderwrack (Fucus vesiculosus), 15 mg (DV not established)

* Irish Moss (Chondrus crispus), 40 mg (DV not established)

* Calcarea fluorica (potentized), 4X (DV not established)

* Lycopus virginicus (potentized), 4X (DV not established)

Thyrostim

Very gentle, Thyrostim is more like a multivitamin for the thyroid. It rarely causes the body to go too fast. If anything, it can take longer and require higher doses. This is best for patients who have a tendency to be sensitive to metabolic stimulation.

Ingredients:

* Vitamin A palmitate, 2,500 IU

* Iodine (from kelp), 150 mcg

* Magnesium, 100 mg

* Selenium (from vegetable), 50 mcg

* Copper, 1 mg

* Manganese, 2 mg

* Rubidium (from vegetable), 25 mcg

* Lamb neonatal pituitary/hypothalamus complex concentrate (from bovine), 40 mg

* Lactobacillus acidophilus (DDS-1), 2 million

* Tyrosine, 100 mg

* Tyrosinase (from mushroom), 10 IU

Medastim

This product is formulated to help patients whose thyroids make plenty of T4 but whose bodies struggle to convert it to T3.

Ingredients:

+ Vitamin B$_1$ (as thiamin mononitrate), 2 mg

+ Vitamin B$_2$ (as riboflavin), 2 mg

+ Niacin (as niacinamide), 20 mg

+ Vitamin B$_6$ (as pyridoxine HCI), 2.4 mg

+ Iodine (from kelp and bladderwrack), 67 mcg

+ Zinc (as zinc gluconate), 4 mg

+ Selenium (as selenomethionine), 30 mcg

+ L-aspartic Acid, 175 mg

+ L-glutamic Acid, 100 mg

+ Glutathione (Reduced), 20 mg

+ L-tyrosine, 100 mg

+ Rubidium (from vegetable culture), 10 mcg

+ Salvia officinalls (leaf), 15 mg

+ Parietaria diffusa (whole herb), 20 mg

Thyrosol

This is a very unusual product because of its ingredients. It contains nothing unique that cannot be found in other thyroid supplements, except for the rosemary leaf. Most descriptions of the benefits of rosemary leaf extract say nothing about its ability to promote thyroid function. Yet Thyrosol works best for certain cases of hypothyroidism.

Ingredients:

+ Vitamin A (as retinyl palmitate), 3,000 IU

+ Vitamin D (as cholecalciferol), 400 IU

+ Vitamin E (as d-alpha tocopheryl succinate), 100 IU

+ Riboflavin, 3 mg

+ Niacin (as niacinamide), 4.5 mg

+ Iodine (as potassium iodide), 76 mcg

+ Zinc (as zinc glycinate), 10 mg

+ Selenium (as selenomethionine), 150 mcg

+ Rosemary Leaf Extract (Rosmarinus officinalis), 79 mg

GTA

GTA is a glandular plus a few minerals.

Ingredients:

+ Porcine thyroid glandular, 5 mg

+ Selenium, 5 mcg

+ Rubidium, 5 mcg

GTA Forte

GTA Forte is a glandular plus a few more minerals.

Ingredients:

+ Zinc gluconate, 10 mg

+ Selenium, 26 mcg

+ Copper gluconate, 1 mg

+ Rubidium, 5 mcg

+ Porcine glandular, 20 mg

GTA Forte II

GTA Forte II is identical to GTA Forte except it contains one-fourth the amount of copper—for patients who are prone to problems stemming from excess copper.

Ingredients:

+ Zinc gluconate, 10 mg

+ Selenium, 26 mcg

+ Copper gluconate, 0.25 mg

+ Rubidium, 5 mcg

+ Porcine glandular, 20 mg

The A-B-Cs of Calcium

People who need to eliminate dairy products from their diets because of an allergy or sensitivity will want to make sure that they consume enough calcium through another source. Is Tums a good source? Is Caltrate good? Both contain calcium in the form of calcium carbonate. So do other supplements—you can tell by checking for "calcium carbonate" on the label.

The following are the best forms of calcium:

+ Calcium chelate

+ Calcium citrate

+ Calcium gluconate

+ Calcium hydroxyapatite

+ Calcium malate

+ Calcium orotate

The following are less-absorbable forms of calcium:

+ Bone meal

+ Calcium carbonate

+ Coral calcium

+ Dolomite

Nondairy and non-grain sources of calcium

One 8-ounce glass of milk contains about 300 mg of calcium, and one ounce of cheddar cheese contains 200 mg of calcium. But people who have eliminated both dairy products and grains from their diets need to obtain adequate calcium from other food sources. The following partial list includes good nondairy and non-grain sources of calcium.[1]

Food	Milligrams (mg) per serving	Percent Daily Value (DV)*
Sardines canned in oil with bones, 3 oz.	324	32
Rice Dream enriched original, vanilla, 8 oz.	300	30
Almond Dream, enriched, unsweetened, 8 oz.	300	30
Almond Breeze, enriched, unsweetened, 8 oz.	300	30
Orange juice, calcium fortified, 6 oz.	200-260	20-26
Tofu, firm, made with calcium sulfate*, ½ cup	204	20
Salmon, pink, canned, solids with bones, 3 oz.	181	18
Blackstrap molasses, 1 Tbsp.	171	17
Tofu, soft, made with calcium sulfate**, ½ cup	138	14
Spinach, cooked, ½ cup	120	12
Turnip greens, boiled, ½ cup	99	10
Almonds, ¼ cup	97	10
Kale, cooked, 1 cup	94	9
Kale, raw, 1 cup	90	9
Soy beverage, calcium fortified, 8 oz.	80-500	8-50
Chinese cabbage, raw, 1 cup	74	7
Broccoli, raw, ½ cup	21	2
Rice Dream, not enriched, 8 oz.	20	2

* Daily values were developed by the US Food and Drug Administration to help consumers compare the nutrient contents among products within the context of a total daily diet. The DV for calcium is 1,000 mg for adults and children aged four years and older. Foods providing 20 percent or more of the DV are considered to be high sources of a nutrient, but foods providing

lower percentages of the DV also contribute to a healthful diet.
** Calcium content is for tofu processed with a calcium salt. Tofu processed with other salts does not provide significant amounts of calcium.

Recommended calcium supplements

I recommend any of the following calcium supplements to patients who come into my office. Calcium absorption is improved with additional vitamin D to increase absorption. (I recommend vitamin D supplementation in the 10,000–50,000 IU/day range.)

- Ca-Zyme (Biotics Research)

- Calcium Citrate (Pure Encapsulations)

- Cal Apatite 1000 (Metagenics)

- Calcimin 300 (Key Company)

- Reacted Calcium (OrthoMolecular Products)

Recommended Books About the Thyroid

Barnes, Broda O. and Lawrence Galton. *Hypothyroidism: The Unsuspected Illness.* HarperCollins, 1976.

Shoman, Mary J. *Living Well With Hypothyroidism: What Your Doctor Doesn't Tell You… That You Need to Know.* Harper Paperbacks, revised edition 2005.

Langer, Stephen and James Scheer. *Solved: The Riddle of Illness.* McGraw-Hill, 2006.

Bowthorpe, Janie A. *Stop the Thyroid Madness: A Patient Revolution Against Decades of Inferior Treatment.* Grape Publishing, 2008.

Shames, Richard and Karilee H. Shames. *Thyroid Power: Ten Steps to Total Health.* Harper Paperbacks, 2002.

Kharrazian, Datis. *Why Do I Still Have Thyroid Symptoms When My Lab Tests Are Normal?* Morgan James Publishing, 2010.

Recommended Websites
About the Thyroid

The following websites can both confirm and elaborate on what I have written in this book:

DrLowe.com (www.DrLowe.com)—Dr. John C. Lowe. Metabolic research and consulting for patients and clinicians.

Dr. Rind.com (www.drrind.com)—Dr. Bruce Rind is a holistic physician with both traditional and alternative medical training, board-certified in anesthesiology with additional training in acupuncture, osteopathy, and nutritional medicine.

Mercola.com (www.mercola.com)—Dr. Joseph Mercola. Natural health information articles and health newsletter.

Stop the Thyroid Madness! (www.stopthethyroidmadness.com)— Janie A. Blowthorpe, thyroid patient activist, author, blogger, teacher.

Thyroid.about.com (http://thyroid.about.com)—Mary Shomon has been a strong advocate for hypothyroid patients for many years. Her site is chock-full of great information and references.

Thyroid Science (www.thyroidscience.com)—Dr. John C. Lowe. *Thyroid Science* is an "open-access journal for truth in thyroid science and thyroid clinical practice."

Thyroid-related Internet groups

For those of you who want to take the reins and be empowered to be an advocate for your own health, I encourage you to take a look at some of these Internet groups hosted by Yahoo. On these websites you can post comments or questions, and other sufferers will try to make suggestions based on their own experiences.

The groups below are active at the time of this writing:

Thyroid (http://health.groups.yahoo.com/group/thyroid)— "Thyroid: Open Forum to Discuss Thyroid Disease" is hosted by Mary Shomon, author of several books about the thyroid and an active advocate for thyroid sufferers.

NaturalThyroidHormones (http://health.groups.yahoo.com/ group/NaturalThyroidHormones)—NaturalThyroidHormones is a group set up for natural thyroid hormone users to promote the use of natural thyroid hormones versus synthetic thyroid hormones such as Synthroid and Levoxyl.

Thyroidless (http://health.groups.yahoo.com/group/thyroidless)— Thyroidless (motto: "No More Roid Rage") is set up to help patients before and after they have had their own thyroids irradiated or surgically removed.

NaturalThyroidHormonesADRENALS (http://health.groups. yahoo.com/group/NaturalThyroidHormonesADRENALS)— NaturalThyroidHormonesADRENALS is set up as a companion group for NaturalThyroidHormones (listed above), but this group is meant specifically for people who also believe that they have adrenal dysfunction in addition to low thyroid.

You can find many more thyroid-related internet chat groups if you search. On such sites, people who would never become acquainted otherwise can share similar experiences and learn from each other. Whether or not you have a local doctor who can help you, you should be able to find people who have had similar experiences and who can spare you from making mistakes. I once had a mentor who said, "The most important treatment is the one that doesn't work." But it's time-consuming, expensive, and discouraging to have to find out everything by yourself.

Where to Find
Nutritionally Oriented Doctors

Chiropractors

For a state-by-state, searchable list of chiropractic internists, go to the website of the Council on Diagnosis and Internal Disorders: http://www.councildid.com/10230/index.html

Naturopaths

For a searchable list of naturopathic practitioners, go to the website for the American Association of Naturopathic Physicians, http://www.naturopathic.org

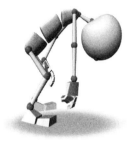

Appendix D

SELECTED PRODUCTS THAT CONTAIN WHEAT AND SOURCES FOR ALTERNATIVES TO WHEAT

This information is also posted on my own website at www.berglundcenter.com/wheat.html. Use this list to increase your grasp of the ingredients included in ordinary foods. If you have a sensitivity to gluten or wheat, you will want to eliminate not only obvious wheat products such as bread made from wheat flour but also some of these products.

Some of the products that may contain wheat

- Breads, buns, and muffins
- Canola oil (similar family)
- Cheeses (processed/mixes)
- Cheerios (added wheat starch)
- Chili (sometimes added as a thickener)
- Chowders (sometimes added as a thickener)
- Cookies

- Cooking spray (some use a grain alcohol, which can be derived from wheat)

- Crackers

- Doughnuts

- Farina (Cream of Wheat)

- Flours (see list below)

- Frozen entrees (always read ingredients list)

- Gravies

- Hydrolyzed vegetable protein

- Pancakes

- Pasta

- Popovers

- Pretzels

- Pringles potato chips

- Salad dressings (some will use or contain food starch or flour for consistency)

- Sauce (use flour as a thickener)

- Vinegar (distilled grain)

- Waffles

Wheat flour and related products

- White flour

- Whole-wheat flour

- Enriched flour

- Wheat starch

- Modified food starch

+ Semolina

+ Durham

+ Graham

Alternatives to Wheat Flour

Here are some companies that sell flourless mixes:

Authentic Foods
1850 W. 169th Street, Suite B
Gardena, CA 90247
(800) 806-4737

This company sells lemon cake mix, vanilla cake mix, chocolate cake mix, cornbread mix, cinnamon bread mix, white bread mix, as well as pancake and baking mix. They also sell a variety of flours, including garfava flour (mix of garbanzo bean flour and fava bean flour), brown rice flour, white rice flour, white corn flour, tapioca flour, potato flour, and potato starch.

Miss Roben's
P. O. Box 1434
Frederick, MD 21702
(800) 891-0083

This company sells a wide selection of bread, cake, cookie, muffin, biscuit, bagel, pizza, and pie crust mixes. In addition, the company sells wheat-free pasta in a variety of styles and also has books for sale.

Ener-G Foods, Inc.
596 1st Avenue S.
P. O. Box 84487
Seattle, WA 98124-5787
(800) 331-5222
(206) 764-3398 (fax)

This company sells a variety of premade wheat-free and/or yeast-free breads, hamburger buns, hot dog buns, English muffins, brownies, cakes, doughnuts, cookies, crackers, breakfast cereals, soups, and pasta. The company also sells Bette Hagman's "Gluten-Free Gourmet Blend," made with three gluten-free flours, in addition to a wide range of single flours. In addition, the company sells dairy-free beverages and gelatin-free (kosher) Jello mixes.

The Baker's Catalog
P. O. Box 876
Norwich, VT 05055-0876
(800) 827-6836

This catalog sells an electric grain mill to make your own fresh milled flour (which is nutritionally superior to anything you can purchase in the store). The catalog also contains a large variety of highly specialized kitchen products.

Cybros Inc.
P. O. Box 851
Waukesha, WI 53187-0851
(800) 876-2253 (876-BAKE)

This company sells a variety of premade breads with and without wheat.

The Gluten Free Cookie Jar
P. O. Box 52
Trevose, PA 19053
(215) 355-9403

This company sells a variety of premade breads, rolls, bagels, scones, cakes, doughnuts, pretzels, and cookies. Mixes are available for muffins, pancakes, breads, and cookies.

Bob's Red Mill Natural Foods, Inc.
5209 SE International Way
Milwaukie, OR 97222
(503) 654-3215
(503) 653-1339 (fax)

Bob's Red Mill Natural Foods catalog lists thirty-one pages of grains, beans, flours, and other baking ingredients. Many of the products are available in grocery stores.

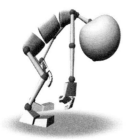

Appendix E

"EATING CLEAN"— SELECTED RECIPES AND TIPS

These recipes and suggestions for "eating clean" have also been collected on my website (www.berglundcenter .com/cooking.html), and I encourage my patients to submit new ones. The recipes have been listed in alphabetical order.

Recipes

Almond (or any nut) Butter Recipe

This is a great recipe for those who are sensitive to peanut butter and can't afford the other nut butters available in grocery stores.

12 oz. raw almonds (or any raw nut)
Extra-virgin olive oil, to desired consistency
Sea salt, to taste

Fill food processor ¾ full with almonds (or other type of nut) and process until powdery. Add olive oil and process until somewhat creamy. (Nut butter will be somewhat grainy.) Add salt to taste. Store in refrigerator.

For a great snack (or breakfast), spread nut butter over Ezekiel 4:9 Cinnamon Raisin Bread. Add sliced bananas and drizzle with honey.

Apple Butter

> 1 lb. tart cooking apples (about three, such as Granny
> Smith), peeled and chopped
> 1 orange
> 1 lemon
> 2 tsp. brown or maple sugar or honey
> ½ tsp. vanilla
> 1 cup apple juice
> ⅛ tsp. ground cinnamon
> ⅛ tsp. ground allspice
> Dash of salt

Place apples in a large, heavy-bottomed saucepan. Remove a 3-inch long strip of peel from the orange and the lemon and add it to the apples. Squeeze the juice from the orange and the lemon; add the juice to the pan. Add remaining ingredients.

Bring mixture to a boil, cover, and cook over low heat for 15 minutes. Uncover and continue to cook over very low heat until mixture is thick—about 45 minutes. The liquid will have evaporated, so stir almost continuously during the final 15 minutes of cooking.

After cooking over low heat for 15 minutes, either place mixture in an oven-proof dish and bake at 300°F, stirring every 10 minutes or so until liquid is evaporated, *or* place mixture in a Crock-Pot and cook all day. Cool mixture to room temperature.

For extra-smooth apple butter, work the apple butter through a food mill or a sieve, or puree it in food processor. Refrigerate in airtight container for up to one week. Makes one cup.

Apple Crisp

> Sliced apples (to fill a 9" x 13" baking dish half full)
> 1 cup rolled oats
> 1 cup Sucanat
> 1 Tbsp. unbuffered vitamin C (ascorbic acid) powder
> ¾ cup oat flour

2½ Tbsp. cinnamon
1 stick butter
Nutmeg (optional, to taste)

Preheat oven to 350°F. Slice apples and fill a 9" x 13" baking dish half full. Sprinkle with ½ cup Sucanat and the vitamin C powder. In a separate bowl, mix remaining Sucanat, rolled oats, oat flour, cinnamon, butter, and nutmeg (if using). Put topping over apples and cook at 350°F for 45–60 minutes until mixture is bubbly and apples are soft (test with a fork.)

Baked Penne[2]

12 oz. Tinkyada brown rice penne
¾ lb. thin asparagus, trimmed and cut into 2-inch pieces
Olive oil cooking spray
¾ lb. lean ground turkey
3 cups tomato sauce
½ tsp. dried basil
¼ tsp. garlic powder
¼ tsp. sea salt
Black pepper, to taste
4 oz. raw cheese, grated

Preheat oven to 350°F. Bring a large pot of water to a boil and cook pasta according to package directions. (Undercook the pasta slightly for best results.) When one minute from being done, add asparagus and boil for one minute; drain and return to pot.

Meanwhile, coat a large skillet with cooking spray and heat to medium-high; add turkey and cook, stirring often, until lightly browned, or about 7 minutes. Add tomato sauce, basil, garlic powder, salt, and pepper, and simmer until heated through, 3 to 4 minutes.

Add turkey meat sauce to penne and asparagus and stir to combine.

Lightly coat a two-quart baking dish with cooking spray; add penne mixture and bake for 18 to 20 minutes. Remove from oven and top with raw cheese. Garnish with oregano or basil if desired.

Banana Bread (brown rice flour)

3 ripe bananas
½ cup honey or 1 cup xylitol
2 eggs
2 cups brown rice flour
2½ tsp. guar gum or xanthan gum
1 tsp. baking soda
¼ tsp. sea salt
½ cup melted butter

In a large bowl, mash bananas until almost smooth. Add rest of ingredients in order and mix thoroughly. Pour into bread pan and bake at 350°F for 50 minutes or until an inserted toothpick comes out clean.

Allow bread to cool until the pan is almost cool enough to touch. Then remove it from the pan. (If the bread is removed too early or too late, it will fall apart.)

Cabbage Soup

1 lb. ground beef, browned
48 oz. V8 or vegetable juice
2–3 cans diced tomatoes
4–5 carrots, chopped
½ package of celery, chopped
6 green onions, chopped
1 yellow onion, chopped
10–15 oz. mushrooms, chopped
½ head of cabbage, chopped
Salt, basil, or other seasonings to taste

Add cooked ground beef to vegetable juice and tomatoes in a slow cooker. Add vegetables. Cook on low for 6–8 hours. Add seasonings to taste.

Chicken and Broccoli With Apricots and Pine Nuts[3]

2 tsp. plus 1 Tbsp. olive oil
4 boneless, skinless chicken breasts
¼ tsp. salt and pepper
1–2 packages of broccoli florets
6 dried apricots, sliced
2 Tbsp. pine nuts (can be omitted)
2 garlic cloves, sliced

Heat 2 tsp. olive oil in a large skillet over medium heat. Season the chicken with salt and pepper. Cook until the chicken is golden brown and cooked through (7–8 minutes per side). Cook the broccoli as directed on the package. Meanwhile, heat 1 Tbsp. of olive oil in a second skillet over medium-high heat. Add the apricots, pine nuts, and garlic and cook, stirring, until the pine nuts and garlic are golden brown (2–3 minutes). Drain the broccoli and add the apricots, garlic, and pine nuts. Serve with the chicken.

Chicken and Sweet Potatoes With Shallots[4]

1½ lbs. sweet potatoes, peeled and cut into 2-inch pieces
2 tsp. salt
4 Tbsp. olive oil
4 boneless, skinless chicken breasts
½ tsp. pepper
4 shallots, sliced into thin rings
2 Tbsp. rosemary

Place the sweet potatoes in a large pot. Add enough cold water to cover and bring to a boil. Add 1 teaspoon salt, reduce heat, and simmer until tender (14–16 minutes). Reserve ¼ cup of the cooking water, drain the potatoes, and return them to the pot. Mash with the reserved cooking water. Meanwhile, heat 1 Tbsp. olive oil in a large skillet over medium heat. Season the chicken with ½ teaspoon salt and ¼ teaspoon pepper; cook until golden brown and cooked through (7–8 minutes per side). Transfer to plates. Wipe out the skillet and heat 3 tablespoons of olive oil over medium-high heat. Add the shallots, rosemary, ½ teaspoon salt, and ¼ teaspoon pepper and cook, stirring, until the shallots are tender (3–4 minutes). Serve the chicken with the potatoes and drizzle with the shallot mixture.

Chicken and Veggie Bake

> 4 chicken breasts
> 1 red bell pepper, cut into 2-inch chunks
> 1 green bell pepper, cut into 2-inch chunks
> 1 can black olives
> 8 oz. fresh mushrooms, sliced
> 1 large yellow onion, cut into 2-inch chunks
> 3 Roma tomatoes, cut into 2-inch chunks
> 3 Tbsp. olive oil
> Dried basil, to taste
> Salt, to taste

Amounts of each of these ingredients can vary depending on taste preference or the number of servings desired.

Cut up the chicken breasts into chunks. Place chicken and all of the vegetables in a 9" x 13" baking dish. Mix in olive oil, basil, and salt. Bake at 350°F for 50–60 minutes.

Chicken Soup

> 2–3 chicken breasts
> 1 large yellow onion
> 1 bunch of celery

1 small package of baby carrots
1 8-oz. package of mushrooms
1 carton of organic, free-range chicken stock
1 large can diced tomatoes
3 bay leaves
Dried basil, to taste
Parsley, to taste
Salt, to taste

Boil chicken breasts in a large pot. Cut up vegetables and mushrooms, and place in a large soup pot with chicken broth. Add diced tomatoes and bay leaves. Once chicken is done, cut into chunks and place in soup pot. Save the water and add as much of it as needed to fill the soup pot. Add basil, parsley, and salt to taste. Simmer until vegetables are cooked. Also can be prepared in a Crock-Pot.

Chicken With Acorn Squash and Tomatoes[5]

1 small acorn squash, halved, seeded, and sliced ¼-inch
    thick
1 pint grape tomatoes, halved
4 cloves garlic, sliced
3 tsp. olive oil
1 tsp. salt
½ tsp. black pepper
4 boneless, skinless chicken breasts
½ tsp. ground coriander
2 Tbsp. fresh oregano, chopped

Heat oven to 425°F. In a large jelly roll pan, toss the squash, tomatoes, and garlic with olive oil, ½ teaspoon salt, and ¼ teaspoon pepper. Season the chicken with the coriander, ½ teaspoon salt, and ¼ teaspoon pepper. Roast everything until the squash is tender and chicken is cooked through, about 20–25 minutes.

Chili

    2–3 lbs. ground beef or ground turkey
    1 yellow onion, diced
    1–2 cans dark red kidney beans
    1 large can crushed tomatoes
    1 large can diced tomatoes
    1 large can tomato sauce
    1 12-oz. can tomato paste
    1 Tbsp. basil
    1 Tbsp. oregano
    ⅓ jar of chili powder
    2 tsp. onion powder
    2 tsp. garlic powder
    Water, to desired thickness
    Salt, to taste

Brown meat and diced onion in a five-quart Dutch oven until the meat is cooked and the onion is soft. Drain fat. Add other ingredients. Simmer and add additional chili powder if desired. This will provide a lot of leftovers. (Also cooks well in a slow cooker.)

Energy Bars

    1 egg
    ½ cup Sucanat
    1 tsp. vanilla
    1 cup granola (see recipe below)
    ½ cup raisins
    ½ cup chopped almonds
    ½ cup dried apricots

Combine ingredients and spread mixture in a greased 8" x 8" pan. Bake for 25 minutes at 350°F. Cool completely before slicing and storing.

Ezekiel Garlic Breadsticks

This is a great alternative to traditional breadsticks.

¼ cup butter
Garlic salt, to taste
2–3 slices Ezekiel 4:9 Bread
Salt, to taste

Melt butter and sprinkle with garlic salt. Cut bread into strips with a pizza cutter. Brush butter and garlic over Ezekiel bread, lightly salt, and bake for 15 minute at 350°F or broil for 1–2 minutes. Great for dipping in organic pasta sauce.

Ezekiel Tortilla Pizzas

This is a great alternative to traditional pizza, but without the wheat or corn syrup.

1 Ezekiel 4:9 tortilla
Organic tomato paste, enough to cover tortilla
1 cup organic chicken, turkey, or beef, chopped and browned
1 cup black olives, onions, green pepper, or your favorite veggies
¼ tsp. oregano
Raw Monterrey Jack cheese, shredded, enough to cover the top of your pizza

Bake an Ezekiel 4:9 tortilla by itself on a cookie sheet for 5–10 minutes at 350°F until somewhat crispy, then top with tomato paste, meat, vegetables, and oregano. Bake the whole pizza for another 10–15 minutes at 350°F. Add shredded raw cheese once the pizza is done baking, and allow it to melt over the hot pizza. Makes one individual pizza.

Fennel-Seed-Crusted Chicken With Roasted Vegetables[6]

¾ lb. carrots, peeled and cut into 3-inch sticks
1 medium red onion, cut into ½-inch wedges
2 Tbsp. plus 2 tsp. olive oil
1 tsp. salt
½ tsp. pepper
4 boneless, skinless chicken breasts
Fennel seeds
¾ cup apple cider
2 tsp. honey

Heat oven to 400°F. In a large jelly roll pan, toss the carrots, onion, 2 tablespoons olive oil, ½ teaspoon salt and ¼ teaspoon pepper. Roast for 20 minutes. Meanwhile, season the chicken with ½ teaspoon salt and ¼ teaspoon pepper, and coat with fennel seeds. Heat 2 teaspoons olive oil in a large skillet over medium-high heat. Cook the chicken, turning occasionally, until browned on all sides (6–8 minutes per side). Transfer the chicken to the pan with the vegetables and roast until the chicken is cooked through and the vegetables are tender (16–20 minutes or more). Let the chicken rest before slicing. Meanwhile, in a small saucepan, combine the cider and honey. Boil until reduced by half (4–6 minutes). Serve over the chicken and vegetables.

Fruity Chicken Salad

1 mango, fresh, sliced
1 package raw spinach leaves
1 package strawberries, fresh, sliced
2 cups red grapes, halved
¼ red onion, sliced
2 avocados, sliced
2 cups organic chicken, cooked and seasoned with olive oil and salt
1 lime
Sea salt, to taste

While slicing up the mangos, squeeze a few slices to obtain 1 tablespoon of mango juice per serving of salad. Top a bed of spinach with sliced mangoes, sliced strawberries, halved red grapes, sliced red onion, sliced avocado, and chicken. Drizzle salad with lime and mango juice. Salt to taste.

Granola

> 5 cups oats
> 1 cup sunflower seeds
> 1–2 cups ground raw almonds
> 1 cup extra-virgin olive oil
> 1 cup honey
> 1 tsp. vanilla

Preheat oven to 350°F. Combine dry ingredients. Add liquid ingredients until granola is moist and stuck together. Spread granola mixture thinly onto jelly roll pans. Bake at 350°F for 25–35 minutes, rotating pans and stirring granola every five minutes. Cool completely before storing.

Granola (alternate recipe)

> 1 cup rice or oat bran
> 1 cup sesame seeds
> 1 cup sunflower seeds
> 1 cup ground walnuts
> 1 cup ground almonds
> 1 cup ground pecans
> 5 cups rolled oats
> 1 cup oil
> 1 cup maple syrup
> 1 Tbsp. vanilla

Preheat oven to 350°F. Combine dry ingredients. Add liquid ingredients until granola is moist and stuck together. Spread granola mixture thinly onto jelly roll pans. Bake at 350°F for 8–10 minutes. Cool completely before storing.

Green Bean Stir-Fry

    1 bunch green onions, cleaned and finely sliced
    Olive or sesame oil
    1 clove of garlic, peeled and diced fine
    2 cups green beans (fresh or frozen)
    2 cups grape or cherry tomatoes, halved (or regular
        tomatoes cut into chunks)
    2 chicken breasts, cooked and cubed
    Sliced almonds

Sauté the onions in the olive oil until soft. Add garlic. Cook two minutes longer. Add green beans and tomatoes; cook until beans are heated through. Add chicken and cook until chicken is browned and pieces are white when sliced open. Just before serving, add the almonds.

Molten Lava Cake

    Olive oil cooking spray
    ¼ cup plus 1 Tbsp. unsweetened cocoa powder
    ⅓ cup Sucanat
    6 Tbsp. unsweetened applesauce
    3 Tbsp. olive oil
    1 egg
    1 egg white
    4 Tbsp. xylitol
    ½ cup spelt flour
    1 tsp. pure vanilla extract
    Strawberries and/or Wax Orchards fudge sauce for
        garnish (optional)

Preheat oven to 400°F. Lightly spray four 4-ounce custard cups or small ramekins with cooking spray. In a medium bowl, combine cocoa powder and Sucanat; whisk in applesauce and oil. In a small bowl, lightly whisk egg and egg white and add to cocoa mixture, whisking until smooth. Add xylitol and mix. Stir in spelt flour and vanilla until flour is combined completely; do not overmix. Divide mixture evenly among prepared custard cups or ramekins, place on a baking sheet, and bake for 9 minutes. Centers should be soft but sides firm. Bake for an additional 1–2 minutes at a time if the centers are still too liquid. Invert the cups onto serving plates; let stand a few minutes before removing cups. Garnish each cake with strawberry slices and drizzle with fudge sauce, if desired, and serve warm.

Oatmeal Crust

> 1¼ cups oat flour
> ¼ tsp. salt
> 2 Tbsp. vegetable oil
> 4–4½ Tbsp. water

Preheat oven to 350°F. Oil a 9-inch pie plate. In a medium-sized bowl, stir together all ingredients with a fork. Pat dough into prepared pie plate. Press pastry between fingers to make an edge. Use fork to prick bottom in several places to prevent buckling. Bake 18–20 minutes or until crust is golden.

Oatmeal-Raisin Cookies

> ¾ cup butter, softened
> ¾ cup xylitol
> ¾ cup Sucanat
> 2 eggs
> 1 tsp. vanilla extract
> 1¼ cups spelt flour
> 1 tsp. baking soda
> ¾ tsp. ground cinnamon
> ½ tsp. salt

2¾ cups rolled oats
1 cup raisins

Preheat oven to 375°F. In a large bowl, cream together butter, xylitol, and Sucanat. Beat in the eggs and vanilla until fluffy. Stir together spelt flour, baking soda, cinnamon, and salt. Gradually beat into butter mixture. Stir in oats and raisins. Drop by teaspoonfuls onto ungreased cookie sheets. Bake 8–10 minutes, or until golden brown. Cool slightly and remove from sheet to cooling rack. Cool completely.

Pancakes (spelt flour)

2 cups spelt flour
1 tsp. baking powder
½ tsp. salt
3 Tbsp. oil (any will do)
2 eggs
1½ cups rice milk, almond milk, or water (to desired consistency)

Mix all ingredients together. Can add rolled oats, nuts, flaxseeds, etc. Cook on a preheated (375°F to 400°F skillet), flipping when bubbles pop, about a minute per side. Pancakes freeze well.

Pasta Fresca

1 package Tinkyada brown rice fusilli pasta
2 Tbsp. olive oil
2 Roma tomatoes, cubed
¼ red onion, sliced
Dash of sea salt and black pepper
½ package baby spinach

Sauce:
¼ cup fresh garlic
2 tsp. salt

¼ cup balsamic vinegar
¼ cup sweet white cooking wine
1 cup olive oil

Cook pasta and drain. Combine olive oil, Roma tomatoes, red onion, salt, and pepper in a large saucepan. Cook until steaming hot. Add baby spinach and cook until just wilted. Combine all "sauce" ingredients and add to the saucepan. Toss with pasta and serve.

Peanut Butter Cookies

½ cup natural peanut butter
1 cup turbinado sugar or Sucanat
2 eggs
1½ tsp. vanilla
1½ cups spelt flour
3 Tbsp. potato flour
1½ cups rice flour
1 tsp. baking powder
1 tsp. baking soda

Preheat oven to 375°F. Cream peanut butter and sugar, then add eggs and whip well. Stir in vanilla. Blend dry ingredients. Mix into egg mixture. Bake 10–11 minutes or until light brown.

Peanut Butter Kisses (spelt flour)

2–4 bars Yamate dark chocolate
1 cup butter
1 cup xylitol or ½ cup honey
1 cup Sucanat
2 eggs
1 cup natural peanut butter
2½ cups organic spelt flour
1 tsp. vanilla
1 tsp. aluminum-free baking powder

1 tsp. baking soda
1 tsp. sea salt
Sucanat or xylitol for rolling (optional)

Break chocolate bars into squares. Cream butter, xylitol (or honey), and Sucanat. Add eggs and beat. Add peanut butter, spelt flour, vanilla, baking powder, baking soda, and sea salt. Roll into 1-inch balls. Roll in Sucanat or xylitol (optional). Place on cookie sheet and bake for 8 minutes at 350°F. Remove from oven. Place 1 chocolate square in the center of each cookie and press down. Bake for another three minutes. Remove from oven and cool completely.

Penne Rosa (dairy free)

1 large clove of garlic
5 Tbsp. olive oil
6 Tbsp. spelt flour
2¼ cups rice milk
1 stick butter
14 oz. Italian diced tomatoes
8 oz. tomato sauce
16 oz. sliced mushrooms (canned OK)
⅓ jar tomato basil pasta sauce
⅔ package frozen chopped spinach (thawed and drained)
Salt, to taste
Red pepper flakes, to taste
1 package Tinkyada brown rice penne pasta

Sauté garlic in olive oil for one minute over medium heat. Add spelt flour and stir for another minute. Add rice milk. Stirring, cook over medium-low heat until thick. Add the stick of butter. Set aside.

Combine diced tomatoes, tomato sauce, mushrooms, pasta sauce, and spinach over medium heat. Add "white sauce" to tomato sauce mixture. Add salt to desired taste. Boil pepper flakes in water and cook Tinkyada brown rice penne pasta according to package directions. Serve sauce over pasta. Add more pepper flakes to desired spiciness.

Pesto (dairy free)

1½ cup fresh basil leaves
2–3 garlic cloves
½ tsp. sea salt
Small handful of raw almonds
5 Tbsp. extra-virgin olive oil

Put all ingredients in a food processor. Process until almonds and basil are finely chopped. Toss with cooked gluten-free pasta.

Pineapple Bread (spelt flour, no eggs)

½ cup applesauce
½ cup melted butter
½ cup honey or 1 cup xylitol
1¼ cups crushed pineapple with juice
1 tsp. vanilla extract
2½ cups spelt flour
3⅛ tsp. baking powder
½ tsp. baking soda
¾ tsp. sea salt
½ cup chopped almonds
Cinnamon for topping
Sucanat or xylitol for topping

Preheat oven to 350°F. Combine applesauce, butter, honey (or xylitol), pineapple, and vanilla. In a separate bowl, combine spelt flour, baking powder, baking soda, sea salt, and chopped almonds. Add dry ingredients to pineapple mixture. Place in a large loaf pan. Lightly sprinkle cinnamon and Sucanat (or xylitol) on top of dough. Bake for 50–60 minutes or until toothpick inserted in center comes out clean.

Protein Bars

> 3 eggs
> 1 cup natural peanut butter
> 1 cup Sucanat
> 2 tsp. vanilla extract
> 1 cup spelt flour
> 4 Tbsp. protein powder
> 1½ tsp. guar gum or xanthan gum
> ¼ tsp. baking powder
> ½ cup chopped nuts
> A little water
> ⅛ cup xylitol
> Yamate dark chocolate (optional)

Combine eggs, peanut butter, Sucanat, and vanilla; blend well. In a separate bowl, combine spelt flour, protein powder, guar gum (or xanthan gum), baking powder, and nuts. Slowly add dry ingredients to peanut butter mixture until well blended. (Add a little water if necessary.) Spread mixture in a 7" x 11" or 8" x 8" ungreased pan. For added sweetness, sprinkle with xylitol. Bake at 350°F for 30 minutes. Cool and cut into bars. Cool completely before storing. If desired, top with dark chocolate.

Rice Flour Pancakes/Flatbread

> 1 cup brown rice flour
> ¼ tsp. salt
> ¾ tsp. baking soda
> ¾ tsp. cream of tartar or ¼ tsp. pure ascorbic acid crystals
> ⅔ cup cooked brown rice (leftover is fine)
> 1 cup soy, rice, almond, or goat's milk, or lukewarm water
> 1½ Tbsp. oil

Preheat a griddle or two nonstick skillets. Combine ingredients, making a medium batter. Spoon tablespoonfuls of batter onto hot surface. When edges brown and seem dry, turn to cook the other side. Repeat with remaining batter. If batter thickens, add a little more liquid.

Variations: Replace up to a third of the flour with ground nuts or seeds. Add ¼ teaspoon of cinnamon or ½ teaspoon of ginger to the batter. Use up to 2 tablespoons of oil in the batter if the griddle tends to stick, and oil the griddle if necessary.

"Rice Krispies" Treats With Peanut Butter

½ cup natural peanut butter
1 tsp. vanilla extract
Pinch of salt
½ cup brown rice syrup
3½ cups puffed rice

Combine the peanut butter, vanilla, salt, and rice syrup in a saucepan; heat until boiling. Remove from heat and immediately stir in the puffed rice. Spoon mixture into a greased 8" x 8" pan. Press evenly to fill in entire pan. Allow to cool, then cut into squares.

Simple Salmon and Green Beans

2 Tbsp. Olive oil
2 boneless, skinless salmon fillets (per person)
Salt and pepper, to taste
Herbs de provence, to taste
½ package whole green beans (per person)
Lemon juice, to taste

Heat olive oil in a large skillet over medium heat. Season the salmon with salt, pepper, and herbs de provence. Cook the salmon until it turns lighter pink throughout (about 4 minutes per side). Meanwhile, cook green beans according to package directions. Serve with salmon. Add a little lemon to the salmon for extra flavor, if desired.

Smothered Mushrooms[7]

2 large portobello mushrooms, stems and gills removed
½ cup salsa
2 Tbsp. green onions, chopped
2 Tbsp sesame seeds, if desired
⅛ cup raw cheese, grated

Preheat oven to 400°F. Place mushrooms upside down (so that each forms a "cup" rather than a "dome") on a baking tray, and top each with salsa and green onions. Sprinkle with sesame seeds (if desired) and bake for 10–12 minutes. Remove from oven and top with raw cheese.

Snickerdoodles

1 cup butter
1½ cups xylitol
2 eggs
2¾ cups spelt flour
2 tsp. cream of tartar
1 tsp. baking soda
¼ tsp. sea salt
2 Tbsp. xylitol (for rolling)
1 tsp. cinnamon (for rolling)

Heat oven to 400°F. Mix butter, xylitol, and eggs thoroughly. Blend spelt flour, cream of tartar, baking soda, and sea salt in a separate bowl; stir into mixture. Shape dough into 1-inch balls. Stir together 2 tablespoons of xylitol and 1 teaspoon of cinnamon. Roll dough balls in xylitol/cinnamon mixture. Place on an ungreased cookie sheet and bake 8–10 minutes. Allow to cool for at least 5 minutes before removing from cookie sheet. Cool completely on wire rack.

Spicy Sweet Potato Fries[8]

3 medium sweet potatoes, cut into strips
1 Tbsp. olive oil
1 Tbsp. chili powder
½ tsp. cayenne pepper (optional)
¼ tsp. sea salt

Preheat oven to 425°F. In a mixing bowl, combine sweet potatoes, oil, spices, and salt, mixing together until fries are evenly coated. Spread fries out in a single layer on a jelly roll pan. Bake for 25–30 minutes, or until crispy on one side. Turn fries using tongs or spatula and cook for another 25–30 minutes, or until golden brown.

Sunny Apple Sandwiches

Mom's answer to peanut butter and jelly for allergic kids!

¼ cup almond or sunflower butter (from health food store)
2 Tbsp. unsweetened applesauce or apple butter
8 rice flour or spelt flour pancakes (see recipe above)
Sprinkling of sunflower seeds, raw or toasted (optional)
Raw apple slices, thinly sliced

Mix the nut butter and applesauce in a small bowl. Spread each pancake/flatbread thinly with the almond or sunflower butter mixture. Sprinkle four of them with a few seeds for "crunch," if desired, and top with apple slices. Put the remaining four thinly-spread pancakes on top of the apple slices, spread side down. Wrap snugly in plastic wrap for the lunch box.

Variations: Use cashew butter in place of the almond butter. May also either omit seeds or substitute sesame or pumpkin seeds. Substitute other fresh fruits, depending on availability: pear, apricot, peach, nectarine, or banana, each sliced to fit the small sandwich.

Tips for eating
clean (substitutions)

Baking powder without corn

3 Tbsp. baking soda
⅓ cup cream of tartar
⅓ cup arrowroot

Combine all ingredients in a jar. Cover tightly and shake vigorously to mix. Store at room temperature for up to one month. Makes about ¾ cup.

Gluten-Free Flour Blend

3 cups garfava flour
2 cups potato starch
2 cups cornstarch
1 cup tapioca flour
1 cup sorghum flour

Note: If sensitive to potato starch, use 4 cups cornstarch. If sensitive to cornstarch, use 4 cups potato starch. In recipes, this blend will match wheat flour cup for cup.

Nut Milk

½ cup chopped cashews, almonds, or any raw (unroasted)
    nut
2 cups warm water
1 tsp. honey
Dash of vanilla
⅛ tsp. salt
⅛ tsp. xanthan gum

Process all ingredients in a blender until very smooth. Strain through cheesecloth-lined colander and refrigerate in an airtight container for up to three days. Makes about 2 cups.

Wheat flour substitutions

To replace 1 standard dry cup measure of white wheat flour, try these substitutions:

- ✦ 1 cup corn flour (note: not cornmeal)
- ✦ ¾ cup cornmeal fine grind
- ✦ ⅞ cup rice flour
- ✦ ⅝ cup potato flour
- ✦ ½ cup barley flour (not gluten free, only wheat free)
- ✦ 1½ cups rye flour (not gluten free, only wheat free)
- ✦ 1½ cups ground rolled oats (not gluten free, only wheat free)

Using honey or xylitol in baking

In baking, replace 2 cups of sugar with ½ cup of honey. Use xylitol in a 1:1 ratio with sugar.

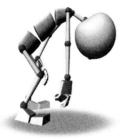

Appendix F

TESTIMONIALS

Many years ago, Dr. Berglund began treating me for injuries sustained from an automobile accident. After realizing that my body was slow to heal, Dr. B. suspected I might have problems with my thyroid. About the same time, I suffered a first-semester miscarriage (my third miscarriage in eighteen months). After reading up and realizing that my miscarriage was a classical example of thyroid-related pregnancy loss, I asked my OB to test my thyroid during routine blood tests. Those test results were "normal," because they were within the lab's accepted levels of 0.5 to 5.5. She said I didn't have thyroid problems.

Dr. Berglund and I really "talked thyroid" after that. My symptoms were a perfect match to those commonly associated with hypothyroidism: extreme sensitivity to cold, low metabolism, unexplained weight gain, thinning hair, skin problems, cold hands and feet, weak immune system, low natural body temperature, difficulty healing, "brain fog," and so forth. He explained to me how the body produces and uses the various "Ts" and how many thyroid medications simply replace missing hormones and ultimately make the thyroid even weaker by taking over its function. He suggested a natural alternative that would help build up my weak thyroid gland. I began to feel much better than I had in years.

A few years later, I saw my regular doctor for a foot injury that could have been a broken bone. During that appointment, we discussed thyroid problems. He did a blood test and formally diagnosed me with Hashimoto's thyroiditis, an autoimmune problem where my body was creating antibodies to fight my thyroid gland. My TSH at that point was in the high 3.0s, but the presence of antibodies suggested I needed medication. He wanted to prescribe synthetic thyroid hormones, because they are more effective and controllable, but I refused to take anything but natural thyroid medication. He put me on a low dose of Armour thyroid.

A year later, when it was time to write a new prescription, my primary care doctor ran another blood test. His office sent me a check-off form that said my results were "normal" and to continue taking my medication. I called in, because I had noticed my symptoms were actually getting much worse and I was also starting to have problems with sudden onset of low blood pressure where I felt like I was going to pass out. I was shocked to learn that the "normal" rating was higher than it had been when I was originally diagnosed, even though I was taking thyroid medication. I asked the nurse to have the doctor increase my dosage based on the blood test results, but he insisted on seeing me in person. He then only increased my dosage by half a tablet more than I was taking. The half tablet increase was almost worse than not taking it. The pills almost disintegrate when you split them, and I had to guess how much of the remaining shards were half a tablet. As a result, my dosage was fluctuating from day to day, and I actually felt worse than I had before.

Prior to the half-tablet increase, I also sought a second opinion from another family practice doctor in the area. He said that I didn't need any additional thyroid medication but suggested that I should be treated for depression based on symptoms like brain fog. This had become a medical nightmare.

I took all this information to Dr. Berglund, who muscle-tested me on my Armour thyroid and his natural alternatives. He said I definitely needed more of both. Knowing my doctor would not be amenable to this, we worked out a plan to use natural alternatives to improve my symptoms along with my current dose of Armour. I don't know where I would be without his wonderful advice and treatment plans. Would anyone have listened to me in the first place and found that my thyroid was, indeed, in trouble? Since the thyroid controls so much of bodily function, would I have been diagnosed with some other problem in the future that was actually the result of reduced thyroid function? Would I be taking potentially dangerous medications that only address certain symptoms and actually cause other problems in the process?

It's funny that doctors who want to "live by the numbers" when it comes to treating thyroid disease are comfortable treating its related symptoms with medications that do not require blood test validation of need or effective treatment levels. I truly don't know where I'd be without Dr. Berglund!

—JENNY

Right after my second child was born, I was *very* tired for a very long time. I'd become sleepy by eight or nine o'clock at night, as I was caring for my young boys. If I had company over or was visiting at relatives' houses, I could not keep my eyes open past 9:00 p.m., even while trying to listen to the fun conversations. I felt I was too young to be so tired.

I even had a housecleaner come to clean my house once a week. The hard part was getting the house ready. It took two hours to pick up the boys' toys so the cleaning lady could clean the house, and after that small task, I was absolutely exhausted.

Then came my first week of teaching the following year. I was feeling dizzy, so I went to have a blood test. The test said my thyroid needed help. So I took the supplement Synthroid for a while. In the meantime, I prayed for a different solution. I also had an aching back; I was getting a pain in my back about every three days.

I come from a family that believed in natural solutions to health challenges. I was directed to Dr. Berglund, who took care of my back through chiropractic care and also through supplements and food choices according to my body's needs. Slowly but surely, my back pain has lessened.

After a while, I asked Dr. B if he could help with my thyroid problem. He said he could, but he could not tell me to stop taking Synthroid, because that would be my choice. I chose to gradually take myself off of the Synthroid and instead to take the supplements he offered. I also chose to make adjustments to my personal diet.

I am currently healthy. I am happy to say that I am no longer on any drugs.

—SHARON

I have suffered from every GI disorder known to man except Crohn's disease (and I wonder about that sometimes too!). At the age of nineteen I was first diagnosed with IBS. I am fifty-two now. I met Dr. B in April of 2007 at a presentation he gave at the public library called, "How Would You Like to Be Medication-Free From Your GI Disorders?" I thought it was impossible, but I was also curious. He really got my attention. I scheduled my first appointment on the spot.

Through the course of the next weeks, I began natural supplements and diet modifications. Before I knew it, we had arrived at a supplemental regimen and diet that suited my system. I could not believe how much better I felt. And I was indeed medication-free for an extended period of time. Dr. B prescribed T-100 for my fatigue and weight gain related to my fibromyalgia and low thyroid. My energy increased, and I even got back to my natural, more comfortable body weight. I seriously believe that without Dr. B's treatment I could not be the active and vivacious woman that I am today.

—TERRI

I was having problems with headaches, stomachaches, and tiredness for some time. The lack of energy really became noticeable after working an eight-hour shift. When I came home, I felt like doing nothing. I didn't want to make dinner, clean the house, or even walk the dog. A family friend recommended Dr. Berglund; she thought he would be able to help. I found out that not only do I have food sensitivities, but I also have an underactive thyroid. I have been tested for thyroid problems in the past, but all the tests came back normal. Dr. Berglund suggested better food choices and taking a thyroid supplement twice daily. After a week, my energy level changed tremendously. I now come home after work with enough energy to take the dog for a walk, make dinner, and enjoy some quality time with my family.

—LAURIE

I have had hypothyroidism for over seven years. Every year my primary medical doctor would increase my levothyroxine in hopes that I would be able to lose weight. My weight never changed. My cholesterol, blood sugar, and blood pressure were sneaking up during this period of time, and my doctor was threatening to put me on medications for all of these things.

As a registered nurse, I have seen people on all of these medications, and I had noted the undesirable side effects. I determined to find a course of action that would address the underlying issues instead of just covering up the symptoms. This is when I decided to see Dr. Berglund. I started on supplements and began to lose weight immediately. I lost an average of one pound a week. When my labs were done again, they showed that my blood sugar was down, along with my blood pressure and cholesterol. I lost thirty pounds over a six-month period. I have lots more energy and feel so much better than I had for years. I have also gone off the levothyroxine medication.

—CHERYL

On my sixtieth birthday I reflected on my life. I realized that for the past six years I had suffered from fatigue and depression, a thirty-pound weight gain, and even a change in personality. After all, I thought, childhood abuse, spousal abuse, and raising three children alone with no financial support were plenty to age me early. Additional stresses included multiple

225

surgeries (hysterectomy, thyroidectomy, skin melanoma surgically removed, and a mastectomy), six prescribed medications, four car accidents, the loss of my job of twenty years, and career change. That was enough stress to feel age ninety instead of sixty, right? No—wrong! This was not acceptable!

Another look back, this time at my family history, made me question my situation, because my seventy-year-old aunt was still mowing her two-acre yard, gardening, and cooking/entertaining groups of a dozen and more people. Another older aunt was driving cross-country. Their life experiences were different from mine, but they too had diseases, families, and stress. What was wrong with me?

After six months of worsening fatigue, I was barely able to continue employment. A friend challenged me to go to a small local gathering because, "You never have any fun anymore." I went. What I found was a brochure of hope—a workshop by Dr. Berglund called "Low Thyroid? Fatigue?" I signed up!

His lecture validated my belief that all my life experiences were connected to my fatigue, but that somewhere out there was the key to recovery. *But*—could Dr. Berglund help someone who not only has low thyroid but *no* thyroid? The line was too long to wait to make an appointment, so I went home.

One Monday morning a week or so after that lecture, I crashed and was unable to go to work. The next morning I was in Dr. B's office for a diagnostic checkup. Medical reports would always say "all is within range" and "her symptoms are vague," but Dr. Berglund took my complaints seriously. His findings were that I was borderline diabetic, showed signs of mercury in my body, my adrenals were taxed, and my thyroid still seemed to be low even though I was taking the conventional synthetic medication Synthroid.

The new prescription was simple: don't eat white enriched flour, sugar, some milk products, and caffeine, and take certain supplements. I continued with the six drugs that had been prescribed—two for high blood pressure, one for depression, one for breast cancer, one for arthritis symptoms, and one for hypothyroidism.

I was faithful to follow the regimen of supplements and diet. Within two weeks I could feel a marked difference. Hope was restored. I lost ten pounds and started wearing a smaller size. My blood pressure returned to normal and then went too low. One by one I declined the synthetic drugs. The arthritis symptoms diminished to just my thumbs, and that could be managed with another natural supplement. My depression declined and could be managed with good rest, good food, and good friends.

Five months after beginning this regimen, I went on a camping trip with my family and participated in tennis, softball, swimming, and water tubing. My daughter said it was like having me back in my thirties. My restored life was nothing short of amazing. At a family gathering, a trip to Dairy Queen was suggested. I replied that I would attend but not partake. Simultaneously my daughters said, "You can have just one cone."

But my son hollered from a nearby room, "Leave her alone! She's finally feeling like people again!"

Now I wake up ready for my day instead of dreading it or in fear that I can't fulfill the tasks ahead. I have the energy to do housework again, participate in church ministry groups, and work a full-time job. I worked many overtime hours in preparation for the last presidential election, and never did that paralyzing fatigue grip me, nor did my blood pressure become alarming.

I take nothing for arthritis pain, and I can open jars, wring out washrags, and lift a gallon of milk. I can run up two flights of stairs, and I walk/run my dog thirty minutes morning and evening.

I feel thirty-something, instead of ninety-something. I know I have found the key for my health.

—LANITA

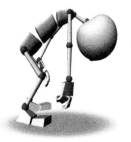

NOTES

Introduction
Helping You Help Yourself

1. Mayo Clinic staff, "Dietary Fiber: Essential for a Healthy Diet," http://www.mayoclinic.com/health/fiber/NU00033 (accessed May 16, 2011).

2. GNC.com, "Top Ten Must Have Supplements," http://www.gnc.com/family/index.jsp?categoryId=4235407 (accessed May 16, 2011).

3. Let me emphasize that legally and clinically I do not prescribe or proscribe. I am a chiropractor by license. Prescribing involves writing a prescription for a patient. Proscribing means taking someone off a medication. My license and training do not include prescribing/proscribing. If I had a patient with high blood pressure, his medical doctor could prescribe drugs to lower his blood pressure. If the same patient came to me, I would try to find out what nutritional deficiency might underlie the high blood pressure. I might see if he would respond to magnesium or L-arginine. I might use his blood pressure as a gauge to see if the deficiencies were being corrected, but I would not be treating his high blood pressure directly. This is an important differentiation. If you are on a prescription medication, a medical doctor or osteopath are the only ones who can legally take you off that medication, or someone else with prescription rights—or you yourself. However, there are risks involved in coming off many medications. A pharmacist can often provide valuable advice.

Chapter 2
Stressed?

1. Based on caffeine contents listed on the website of the Center for Science in the Public Interest, http://www.cspinet.org/new/cafchart.htm (accessed May 16, 2011): Excedrin Extra Strength, 2 tablets, 130 mg caffeine; Mountain Dew, 12-ounce can, 54 mg caffeine; coffee, 8 ounces, 133 mg caffeine.

Chapter 4
Healthy Eating

1. Delta Farm Press, "Monsanto: New Roundup Ready Corn 2 System," October 3, 2003, http://deltafarmpress.com/monsanto-new-roundup-ready-corn-2-system (accessed May 25, 2011).

2. Environmental Health, "Disinfection By-Products (DBPs)," Centers for Disease Control and Prevention, http://www.cdc.gov/exposurereport/pdf/THM-DBP_FactSheet.pdf (accessed May 26, 2011).

3. Ibid.

4. Jeff Donn, Martha Mendoza, and Justin Pritchard, "AP: Drugs Found in Drinking Water," *USA Today*, September 12, 2008, http://www.usatoday.com/news/nation/2008-03-10-drugs-tap-water_N.htm (accessed May 26, 2011).

5. For more information, visit Pure Earth Technologies at their website, http://www.pure-earth.com/pro.html.

Chapter 5
Is Your Thyroid an Underachiever?

1. Section on Clinical Pharmacology and Therapeutics, Committee on Drugs, "Fever and Antipyretic Use in Children," *Pediatrics* 127, no. 3 (March 1, 2011): 580–587; http://pediatrics.aappublications.org/cgi/content/full/127/3/580 (accessed May 26, 2011).

2. Thyrosol is included in the list of recommended supplements in the back of this book. See Appendix C.

3. Alessandro Di Stefani, Augusto Orlandi, Sergio Chimenti, and Luca Bianchi, "Phrynoderma: A Cutaneous Sign of an Inadequate Diet," *Canadian Medical Association Journal* 177, no. 8 (October 9, 2007): 855–856; http://www.ncbi.nlm.nih.gov/pmc/articles/PMC1995140/ (accessed May 26, 2011).

4. B. O. Asvold et al., "Thyrotropin Levels and Risk of Fatal Coronary Heart Disease: The HUNT Study," *Archives of Internal Medicine* 168, no. 8 (April 28, 2008): 855–860; http://www.ncbi.nlm.nih.gov/pubmed/18443261 (accessed May 26, 2011).

5. Salman Razvi et al., "The Beneficial Effect of L-Thyroxine on Cardiovascular Risk Factors, Endothelial Function, and Quality of Life in Subclinical Hypothyroidism: Randomized, Crossover Trial," *Journal of Clinical Endocrinology & Metabolism* 92, no. 5 (May 2007): 1715–1723; http://jcem.endojournals.org/content/92/5/1715.full (accessed May 26, 2011).

6. Mary Shomon, "Fibromyalgia Aches and Pains as a 'Symptom' of Hypothyroidism: Theories of Dr. John Lowe," Thyroid-info.com, April 8,

2011, http://www.thyroid-info.com/articles/drlowefms.htm (accessed May 26, 2011).

7. Ibid. For more information, see also Mary J. Shomon, "The Thyroid/Fibromyalgia Connection: Shared Causes, Shared Treatments?" About.com, May 12, 2004, http://thyroid.about.com/cs/fibromyalgiacfs/a/fibrothyroid.htm (accessed May 26, 2011).

Chapter 7
What Hormones and Substances Inhibit Your Thyroid?

1. E. M. Sunderland, "Mercury Exposure From Domestic and Imported Estuarine and Marine Fish in the U.S. Seafood Market," *Environmental Health Perspectives* 115 (2007): 235–242, as referenced in Whfoods.com, "Should I Be Concerned About Mercury in Fish and What Fish Are Safe to Eat?," http://www.whfoods.com/genpage.php?tname=george&dbid=103 (accessed May 27, 2011).

2. See articles by Dr. Joseph Mercola such as "Why Soy Can Damage Your Health," at http://articles.mercola.com/sites/articles/archive/2010/09/18/soy-can-damage-your-health.aspx.

3. "Bioidentical Hormone Replacement Therapy" courtesy of Chapel Hill Compounding Specialty Pharmacy Services, Chapel Hill, NC, http://www.chapelhillcompounding.com/services/hrt.

4. Ibid.

5. J. E. Rossouw, G. L. Anderson, G. L. Prentice, et al., "Risks and Benefits of Estrogen plus Progestin in Healthy Postmenopausal Women: Principal Results From the Women's Health Initiative Randomized Controlled Trial," *Journal of the American Medical Association* 288, no. 3 (July 17, 2002): 321–333. Also, G. L. Anderson, M. Limacher, A. R. Assaf, et al., "Effects of Conjugated Equine Estrogen in Postmenopausal Women With Hysterectomy: The Women's Health Initiative Randomized Controlled Trial," *Journal of the American Medical Association* 291, no. 14 (April 14, 2004): 1701–1712.

Chapter 8
Tests to Diagnose Thyroid Problems

1. Janie Bowthorpe, "Ferritin, Iron and Hypothyroidism," Stopthe ThyroidMadness.com, www.stopthethyroidmadness.com/ferritin (accessed May 27, 2011).

2. Ibid.

3. Ibid.

4. Regarding iron and selenium deficiency associated with low thyroid, see also M. B. Zimmermann and J. Kohrie, "The Impact of

Iron and Selenium Deficiencies on Iodine and Thyroid Metabolism," *Thyroid* 12, no. 10 (2002): 867–878; http://www.ncbi.nlm.nih.gov/pubmed/12487769?dopt=Abstract (accessed May 27, 2011).

Chapter 9
Resurrecting the Thyroid

1. To learn about some alternatives to Synthroid, go to www.stopthethyroidmadness.com or www.thyroid.about.com. Both of these websites were founded and are maintained by individuals who write as patient advocates.

2. For your convenience, I have set up a site so you can get all the products that I am listing here in this book: www.notmedicine.com.

3. For more information about the connection between anemia and hypothyroidism, see Sonja Y. Hess, Michael B. Zimmermann, Pierre Adou, Toni Torresani, and Richard F Hurrell, "Treatment of Iron Deficiency in Goitrous Children Improves the Efficacy of Iodized Salt in Côte d'Ivoire," *American Journal of Clinical Nutrition* 75, no. 4 (2002): 743–748; http://www.ajcn.org/content/75/4/743.full (accessed June 3, 2011).

Chapter 11
The Body Is Always Right

1. Robert Thom, "Ignaz Philipp Semmelweis (1818–65)," *Emerging Infectious Diseases* 7, no. 2 (March–April 2001): http://www.cdc.gov/ncidod/eid/vol7no2/cover.htm (accessed June 3, 2011).

2. As referenced in The Center for Unhindered Living, "The Dangers of Prenatal Ultrasound," http://www.unhinderedliving.com/pultra.html (accessed June 3, 2011).

Appendix A
Axillary/Basal Temperature Test

1. The Axillary/Basal (Barnes) Temperature Test was developed from Broda Barnes and Lawrence Galton, "The Flaw in Diagnosis...and Overcoming It," in *Hypothyroidism: The Unsuspected Illness* (New York: HarperCollins, 1976).

Appendix B
Artificial Sweeteners

1. Burkhard Bilger, "The Search for Sweet," *The New Yorker*, May 22, 2006, http://business.highbeam.com/410951/article-1G1-146638573/search-sweet (accessed June 3, 2011).

2. Joseph Mercola and Kendra Degen Pearsall, *Sweet Deception* (Nashville: Thomas Nelson, 2007), 98.

3. Japan Food Chemical Research Foundation, "A Report on Sucralose From the Food Sanitation Council," January 6, 1999, http://www.ffcr.or.jp/zaidan/FFCRHOME.nsf/pages/e-kousei-sucra (accessed June 3, 2011).

4. As quoted in Fran Gare, *The Sweet Miracle of Xylitol* (n.p.: Basic Health Publications, Inc., 2003), 17.

Appendix C
Dr. B's Suggestions

1. Office of Dietary Supplements, "Dietary Fact Sheet: Calcium," http://ods.od.nih.gov/factsheets/Calcium-HealthProfessional/ (accessed June 3, 2011). A comprehensive list of all foods containing calcium can be found on the United States Department of Agriculture (USDA) National Nutrient Database for Standard Reference, Release 20, at http://www.nal.usda.gov/fnic/foodcomp/Data/SR20/nutrlist/sr20a301.pdf (accessed June 3, 2011).

2. Adapted from *Clean Eating* magazine, Robert Kennedy Publishing, Mississauga, ON, Canada.

3. Adapted from *Real Simple* magazine, Time, Inc. Home Entertainment, New York.

4. Ibid.

5. Ibid.

6. Ibid.

7. Adapted from *Clean Eating* magazine.

8. Ibid.